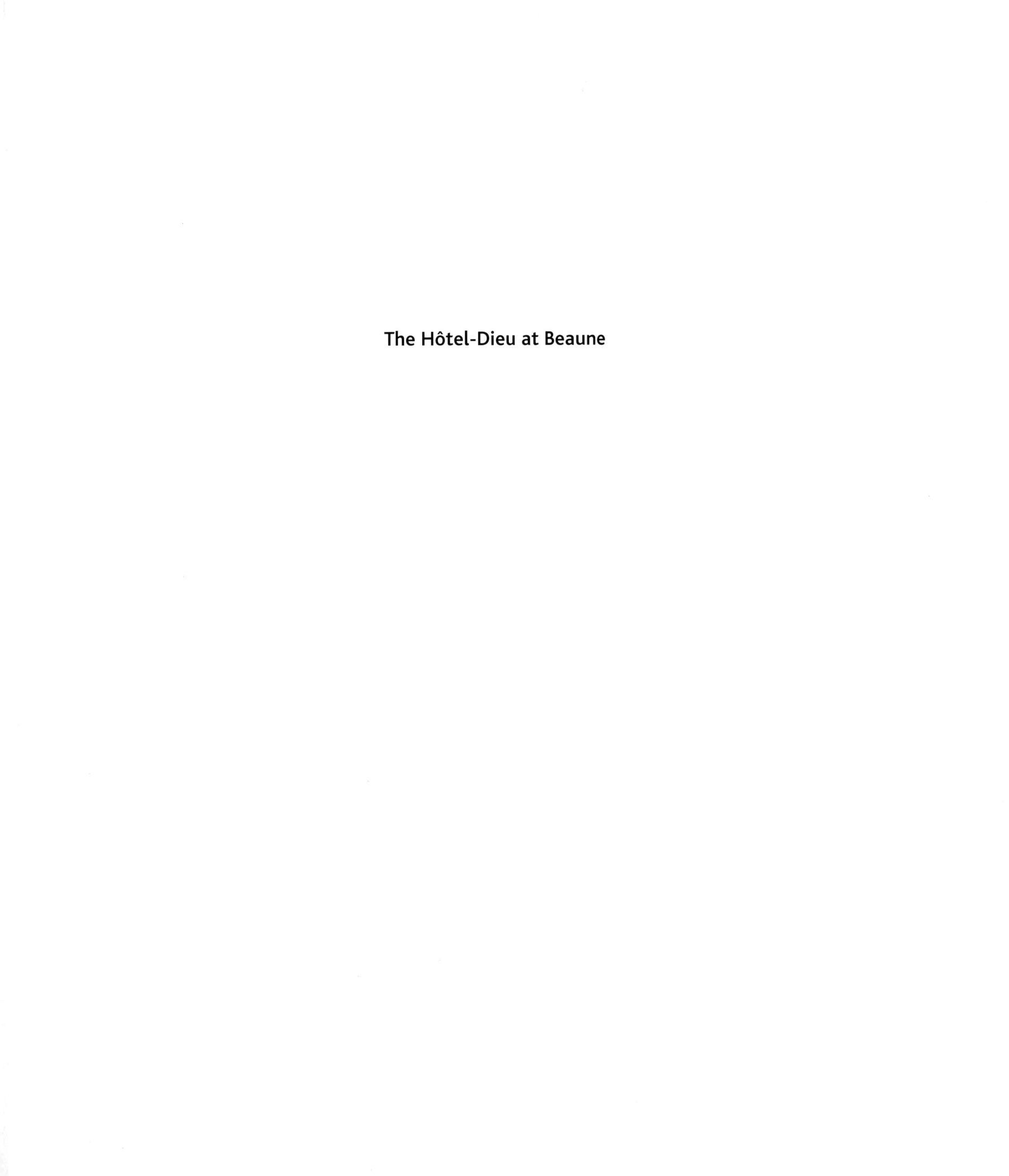

The Hôtel-Dieu at Beaune

© Somogy éditions d'art, Paris, 2005
© DRAC Bourgogne, service régional
de l'Inventaire général, 2005
© Hospices civils de Beaune, 2005

Edited and published by Somogy éditions d'art
Graphic design: Valentina Léporé
Production: Michel Brousset, assisted by Mara Mariano
and Sandrine Arthur
English translation and editing: John Tittensor
Coordinating editor: Isabelle Dartois

ISBN 2-85056-848-1
Legal registration: April 2005
Printed in Italy

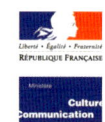

The Hôtel-Dieu at Beaune

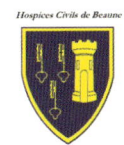

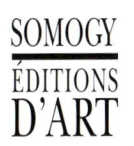

The authors

Articles:
Claudine Hugonnet-Berger, Chief Heritage Curator
Brigitte Fromaget, researcher at the Regional General Inventory (BF)

Élisabeth Réveillon, Chief Heritage Curator (ÉR)

Bruno François, Executive Curator, Antiquities and Objets d'Art (B Fran)

Christine Locatelli, Dendrochronology Laboratory, Department of Archaeology, University of Sheffield, UK

Didier Pousset, Dendrochronology Consulting, Sheffield, UK

Preface by Sylvie Le Clech, Regional Curator at the General Inventory

Photographs:
Michel Rosso,
Jean-Luc Duthu,
Michel Thierry,
photographers at the Regional General Inventory

Maps:
Alain Morelière, consulting engineer

Acknowledgements

For their specialist contributions: Dr Didier Sécula, historian; Christine Locatelli and Didier Pousset, dendrochronologists; Renaud Benoît-Cattin and Pierre Jugie, Regional Curators at the Burgundy General Inventory from 1991 to 2001.

For their kind assistance: the Hospices Civils de Beaune and the staff of the former Hôtel-Dieu.

Contents

Introduction	6
Sylvie Le Clech	
Plan of the ground floor and upper floor	8
Alain Morelière	
History and architecture	12
Claudine Hugonnet-Berger	
Building the Hôtel-Dieu	14
Water	18
Stone	18
Wood	21
▮ Dendrochronology	21
▮ From the forests at Argilly, Borne, Champ-Jarley and Épenôt to the roof structures of the Hôtel-Dieu	22
Christine Locatelli and Didier Pousset	
Slate	27
Clay	27
Metal	28
The evolution of a 15th-century building	30
The Great Hall of the Poor and the chapel	30
The "Infirmary for the grievously ill"	36
The private room	38
The kitchen	45
The ovens and the flour store	47
The refectory cellar	48
The winepress house	49
The laundry and outdoor wash-house	50
From dispensary to pharmacy	50
▮ A mid-18th-century dispensary	53
The nuns' rooms	54
The garden extension and the cemetery	58
Major restoration campaigns	62
Decoration and furnishings	64
Brigitte Fromaget, Élisabeth Réveillon, Bruno François	
The founders and their image (BF)	66
Caring for the soul	68
Rogier Van der Weyden's masterpiece (ÉR)	68
Tapestries and textiles in the chapels (BF)	72
The paintings (BF)	75
▮ An odd picture in the refectory (BF)	79
Devotional statues (BF)	80
Saints and healers (BF)	83
The sacristy (ÉR)	86
▮ The Antoine de Salins bell (BF)	87
Women and men at the service of the sick (BF)	88
The hospitaller nuns (BF)	88
The doctors (BF)	90
The benefactors (BF)	91
Functional furnishings (B Fran)	92
Beds for the poor (B Fran)	92
From chests to cupboards (B Fran)	94
▮ Marking the furniture (ÉR)	98
Care and nourishment (B Fran)	99
▮ The dove tapestries (BF)	101
Everyday items (BF)	102
▮ A rare hospital feeding cup (ÉR)	105
From hospital to museum (ÉR)	106
An impressive tapestry collection (BF)	106
▮ A precious casket (BF)	113
A souvenir of the Clermont-Tonnerre family (ÉR)	114
The bequest of a discerning collector (ÉR)	118
A collection of wine-tasting cups (ÉR)	118
▮ Back to the roots (ÉR)	119
The Hospices de Beaune vineyards	120
The sale of Hospices de Beaune wines	122
The hospital today	124
Bibliography	126

Introduction

The group of buildings making up the Hôtel-Dieu – which now attracts over 400,000 visitors per year – accounts for a large part of what historians and art historians know about hospitals under the Ancien Régime, in all their diversity and their evolution over time. Here lies the explanation for the renown and the emblematic character of a once purely utilitarian institution that achieved heritage status with its restoration in 1872 by Maurice Ouradou, pupil and son-in-law of the most famous of France's Historical Monuments architects, Viollet-le-Duc.

With that restoration the Hôtel-Dieu's public image was established for future generations. Its architecture and interiors had not been "updated", but thoroughly brought into line with the 15th century – or the way that century was imagined at the time. Testimony to the generosity and social conscience of the man who founded it in 1443 – Nicolas Rolin, chancellor to the Duke of Burgundy – the Hôtel-Dieu was to become the symbol of the medieval hospital. And with its multicoloured roofs, it also came to represent Burgundy – even though those tiles, a pure product of a poetic imagination, were only laid in 1902-07.

In other words, a closer look tells us that the story is less simple than it first appears. This book, the work of a team including historians, historians of architecture, decoration and furnishings, and tree-ring dating specialists is intended to bring to light a host of little-known aspects of a building and its contents first presented to the public in 1971, when its original function was taken over by Beaune's new hospital. "List, study and above all, make known": such were the tasks laid down by André Malraux in 1964 when he established France's General Inventory of Monuments and Art Treasures. Setting out with no aesthetic preconceptions and accepting of the inconsistencies and grey areas inherent in a long history, the Inventory's regional teams were determined to use their documentary and artistic expertise, plus photos and architectural elevations, to offer the public all the richness of a heritage under-appreciated because everybody thought they already knew all about it. And so this book offers the reader vital new information on the dating of the Hôtel-Dieu's roof structures, its remarkable collection of medieval chests, and many other historic pieces of which only a small part can actually be displayed. Beaune's Hôtel-Dieu is in a similar situation to other buildings belonging to the Burgundian, national and European heritage: it may never have been celebrated by the poet Verlaine, as was the Broussais hospital in Paris, but setting it in a broader context by comparing it with other hospitals dating from the second half of the Middle Ages gives us a clearer view of its specific features and answers some of the questions it raises.

The Beaune Hôtel-Dieu is part of a corpus of some 600 establishments identified by the General Inventory's regional section in Burgundy's four *départements*. 125 of them have been researched in depth, but only 14 sites ranging from the 12th to the 15th century are still available for study, eight of them in the Côte-d'Or département and five in the Yonne. Equalled only by the Tonnerre hospital in the Yonne, Beaune's is a fine example of the evolution of such institutions in the course of the Middle Ages: beginning as small, scattered establishments — lazarettos, "houses of God", leprosariums — offering shelter and medical care, they comprised a chapel, a single ward and a handful of utility or agricultural buildings. The following phase, the creation of true hospitals, took place in parallel with the arrival of Franciscan and Dominican monasteries in cities and towns between the 13th and 15th centuries.

An architectural landmark in any city, the Hôtel-Dieu was habitually set around a courtyard whose initial nucleus remained visible in the form of little rural buildings: the hall of the poor and the chapel, symbols of the physical and spiritual health that were seen as intimately related in the Middle ages. To the nucleus were added other buildings that more or less expressed the establishment's functioning via their layout and their connection with the hospital area. In addition to the nuns' quarters and the utility rooms in Beaune, and contrary to certain preconceptions about the period, we find the dying isolated in the "infirmary", eight private rooms and very early — a little before 1500 — a dispensary and a library. These were signs that, at the end of the Gothic age, it was no longer enough simply to provide the poor and the sick with shelter in a single, dubiously hygienic ward; now there was a concern with accumulating practical medical skills and scientific knowledge in the interest of improved care. Thus the hospital continued to grow and adapt right through into the 20th century. Of course the hospital of our time is no longer the "house of the sick poor"; economic change has meant that its doors are now open to all classes of society.

A place where the generations mingled and found a sense of community, Beaune's Hôtel-Dieu sums up, in its configuration and its contents, a society that coped with a host of paradoxes from the Middle Ages down to the present: architecture that was at once impressive and utilitarian to the point of starkness; and the contrast between the virtuosity of Rogier Van der Weyden's *Last Judgement* polyptych, the luxurious tapestries, the gold and silver ware, and the humbleness of the domestic items.

Thus we come to understand that the true richness of this building is the profound humanity that emanates from it even today: for this has been a living heritage for over five centuries.

The poet Scarron asserted that there were always enough learned men in the Hôtel-Dieu in Paris to found an Academy. And now that we know Beaune's Hôtel-Dieu in all its diversity, we see that it has nothing to envy its prestigious neighbours.

Sylvie Le Clech
Regional curator of the General Inventory

PLAN OF THE GROUND FLOOR

1 - vestibule
2 - great Hall of the Poor
3 - chapel
4 - sacristy
5 - chambre Sainte-Anne
6 - salle Saint-Hugues
7 - salle Saint-Nicolas
8 - kitchen
9 - boardroom
10 - covered passageway
11 - pharmacy
12 - dispensary
13 - laboratory
14 - salle Saint-Louis
15 - hall of the polyptych
16 - chaplains' quarters
17 - covered passageway
18 - nuns' refectory
19 - head nun's room
20 - the "refectory cellar"

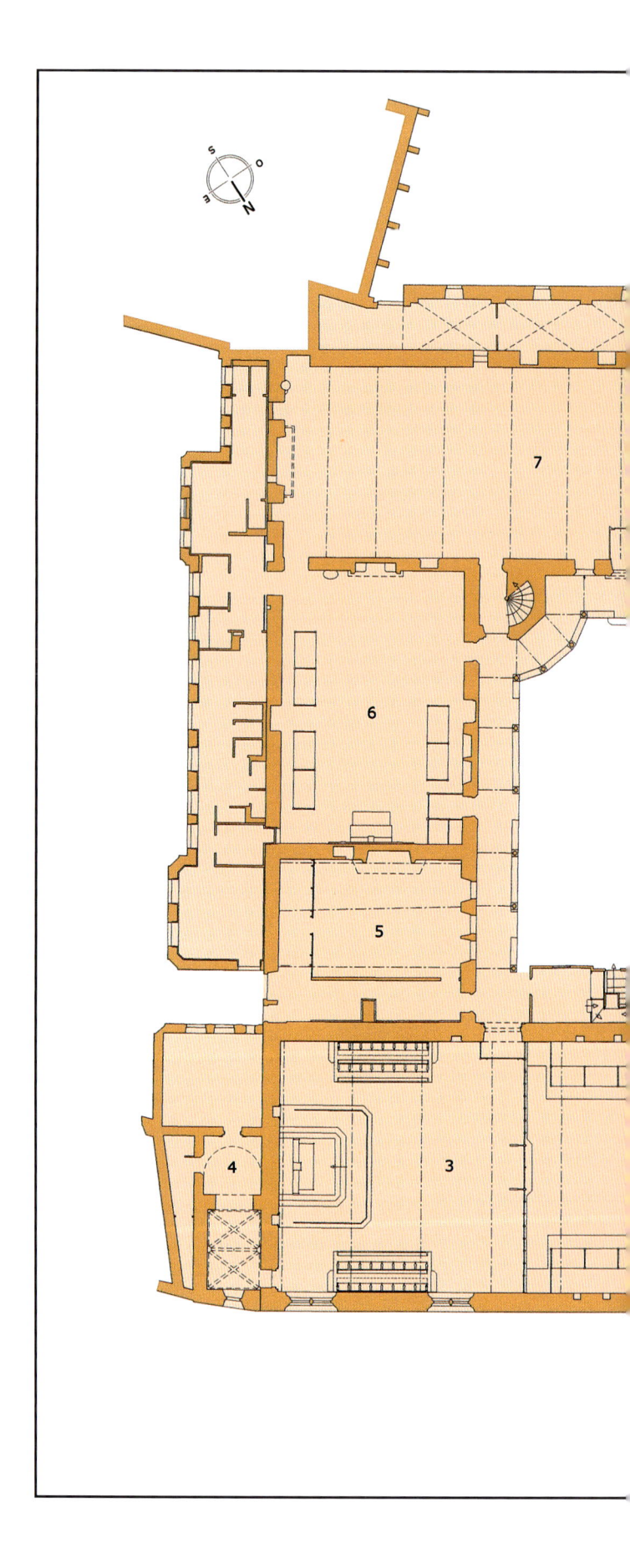

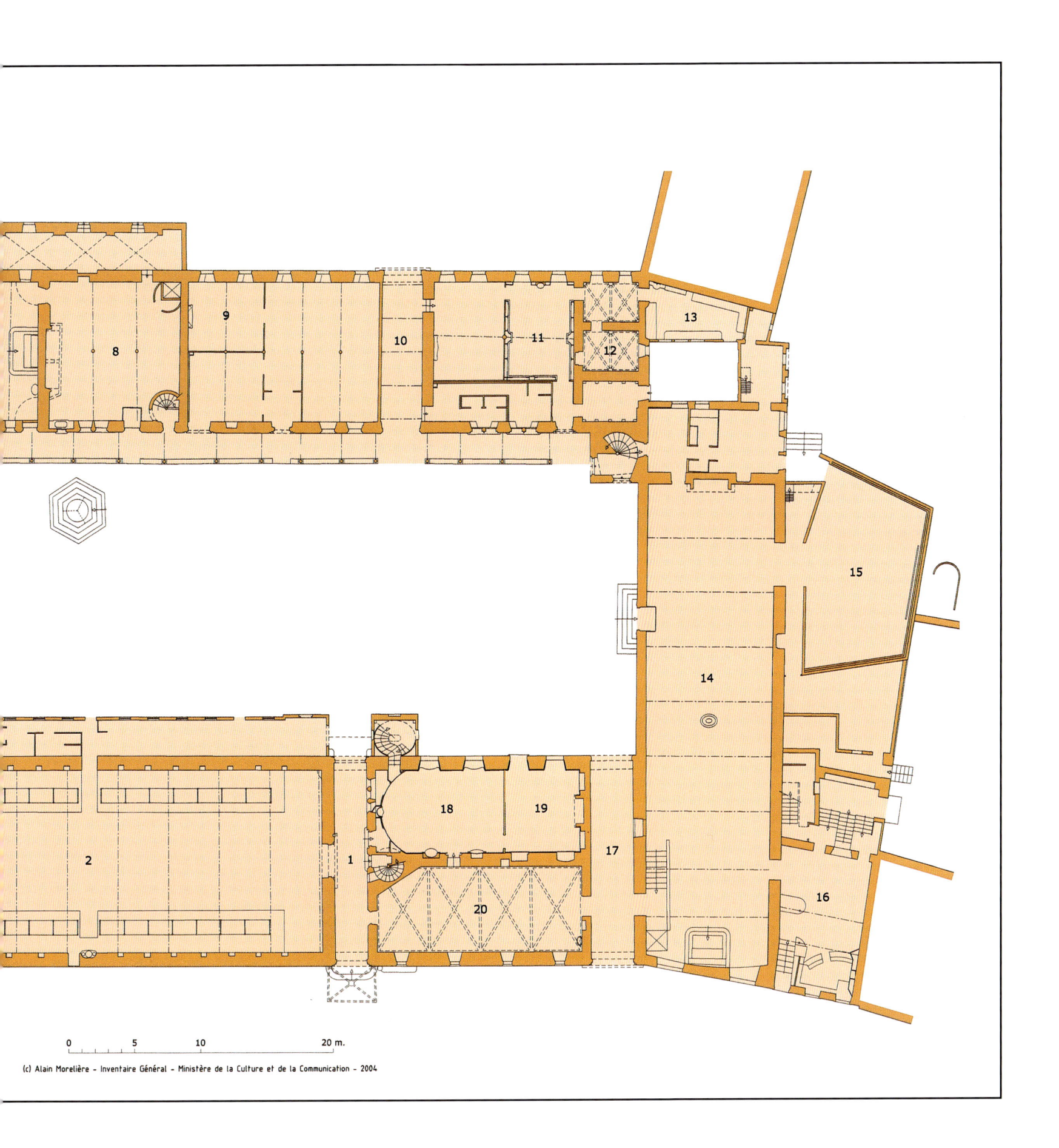

(c) Alain Morelière - Inventaire Général - Ministère de la Culture et de la Communication - 2004

PLAN OF THE UPPER FLOOR

21 - chambre-Dieu
22 - seminar rooms
23 - the King's Room
24 - archives
25 - dovecote
26 - nuns' dormitory

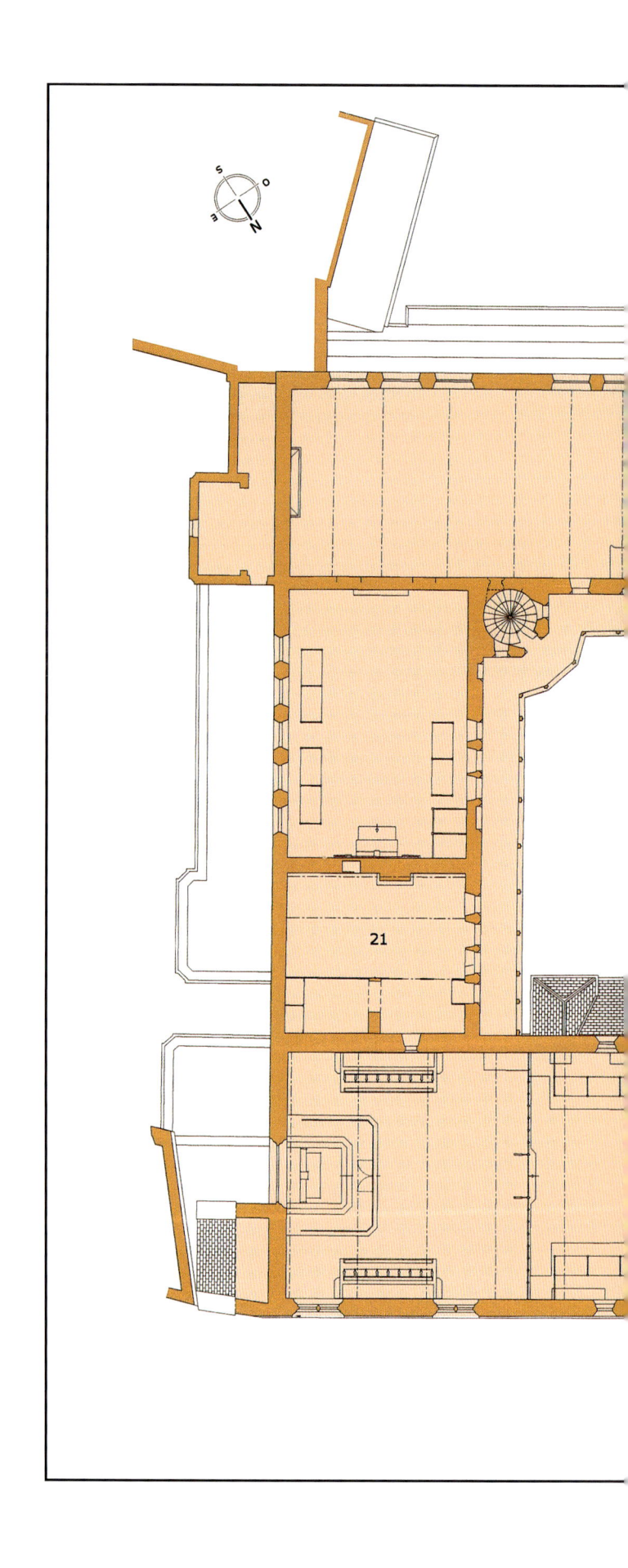

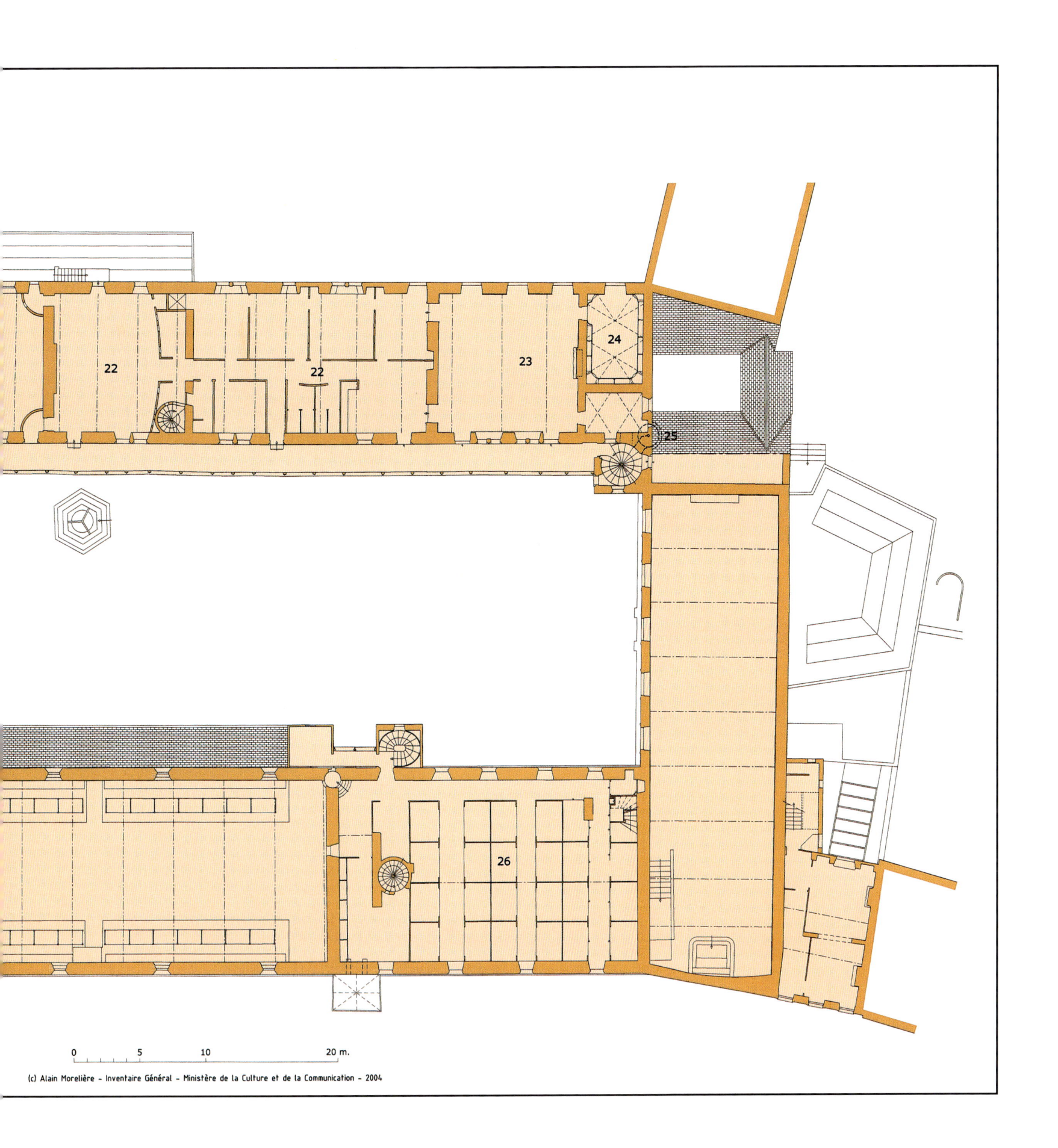

(c) Alain Morelière – Inventaire Général – Ministère de la Culture et de la Communication – 2004

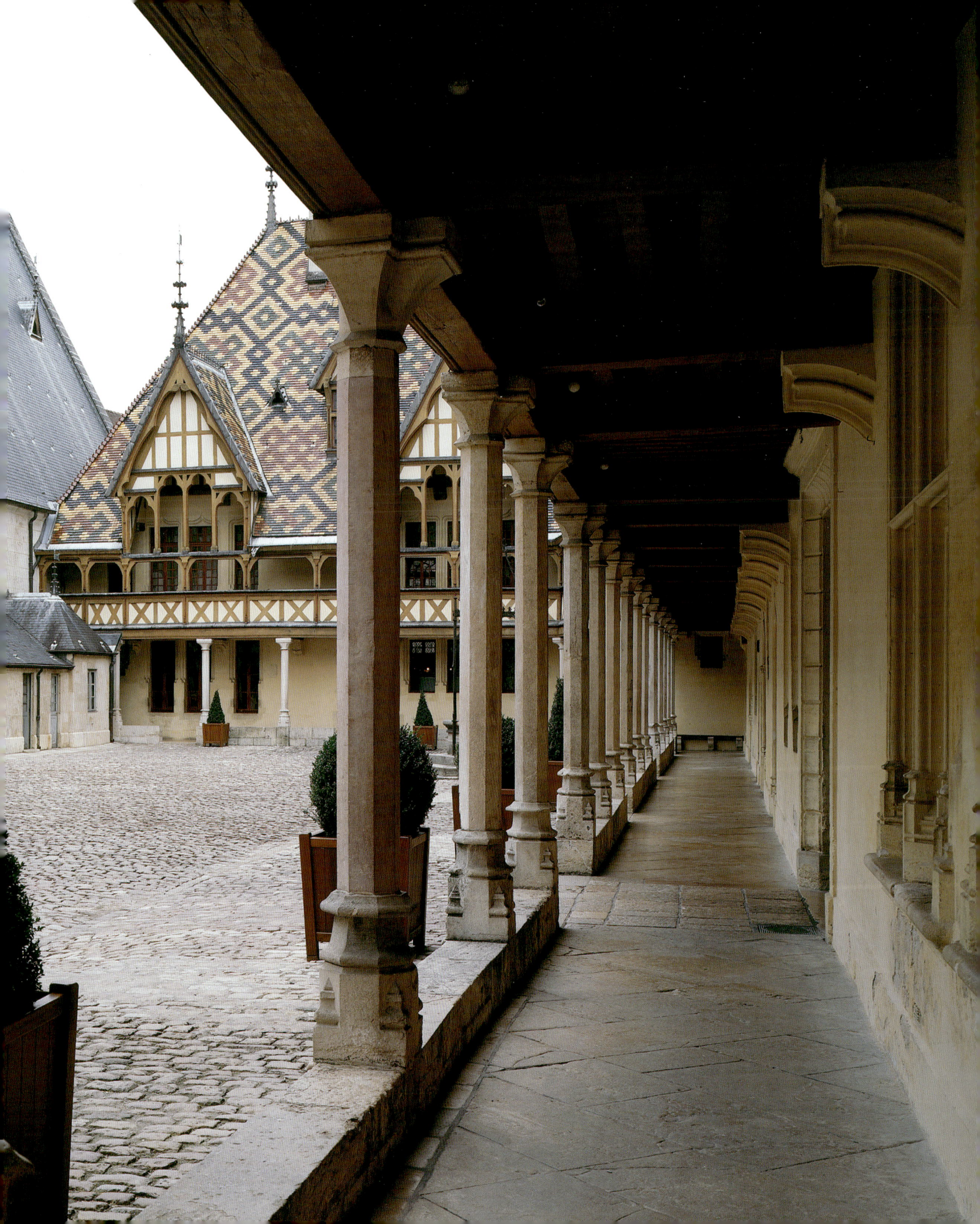

HISTORY AND ARCHITECTURE

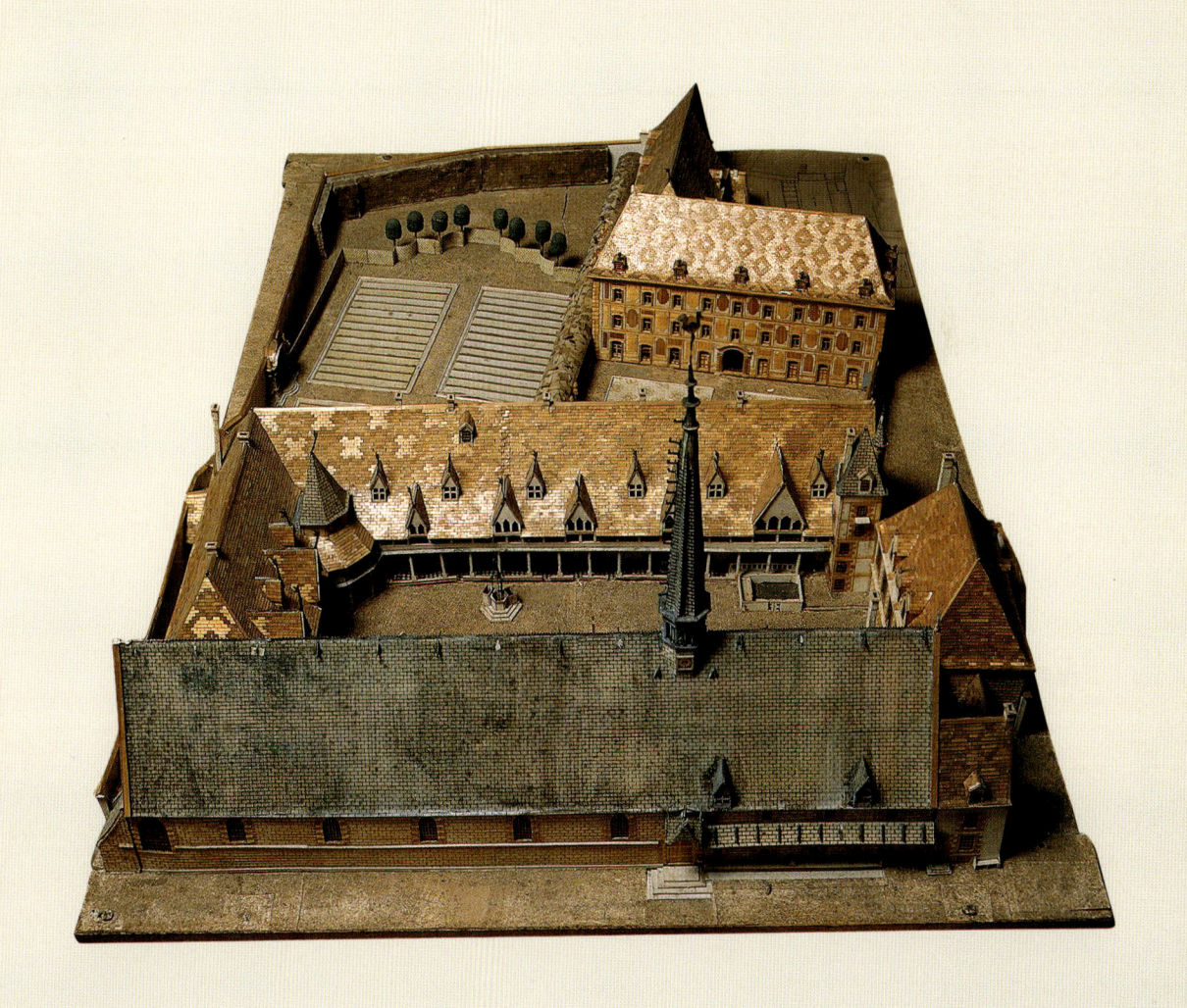

Building the Hôtel-Dieu

The year 1447 was drawing to a close when the first cartloads of slate for the Hôtel-Dieu hospital reached the Place des Halles in the centre of Beaune. Work had already been under way for more than four years: the masonry of the main building giving onto the street was almost finished, the carpenters were busy and the two wings on the courtyard were taking shape. However, the project was taking longer than planned, and Nicolas Rolin, Duke of Burgundy (1376-1462) was not pleased: ageing, and anxious about the after-life, he had insisted that the building process should take no more than four or five years, but an enormous amount still remained to be done. On 4 August 1443, on the forecourt of the collegiate church of Notre Dame, he had read the foundation charter of his hospital to the people of Beaune: to ensure his "personal salvation", King Philip the Good's immensely wealthy chancellor was putting his fortune at the service of "the sick poor". He made no mention of the wretchedness of the common people or of the epidemics and other disasters they had suffered. Nonetheless, the activity generated by this remarkable project was to be an extraordinary force for change in this small city: we need only imagine the impact of such large-scale works on daily life, as carts endlessly came and went and the streets seethed with tradesmen and labourers. Nor was any mention made, despite her manifest involvement, of Guigone de Salins, Nicolas Rolin's third wife: her name figures neither in the charter nor in the Hôtel-Dieu's rules and regulations as drawn up by her husband in 1459. Only Pope Pius II's bull of the same year, confirming the establishment's privileges and statutes, refers to the personal contribution she made.

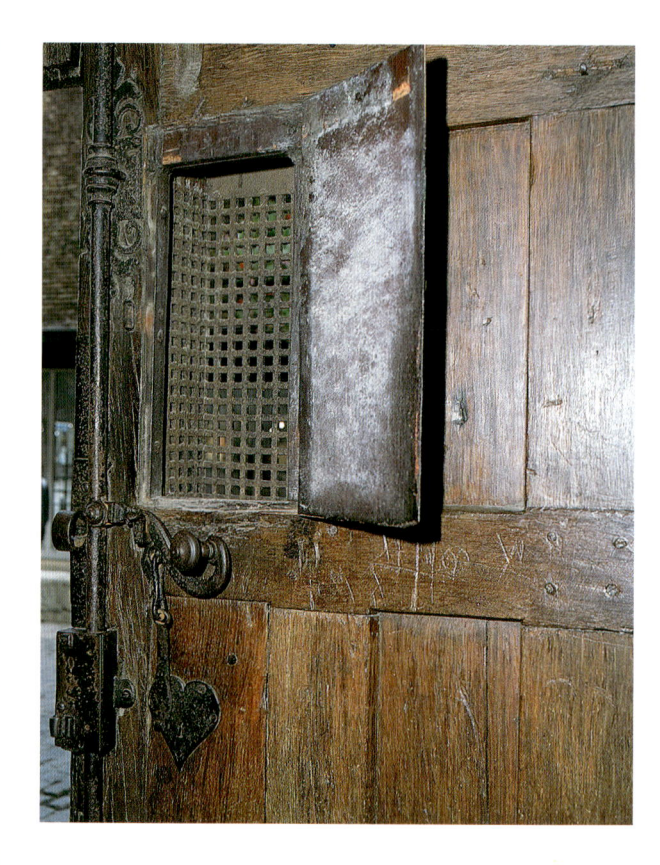

With a handful of exceptions, the architects of the Middle Ages have remained anonymous; and this holds true – apart from a much-contested hypothesis regarding a certain Jacques Wiskerc – for the Hôtel-Dieu in Beaune. All the indications are that the

▌Previous pages:
Left: The lower gallery of the large courtyard wing.
Right: The "straw hospital" model of the Hôtel-Dieu, dating from the mid-17th century.
This page: The spyhole at the entrance.

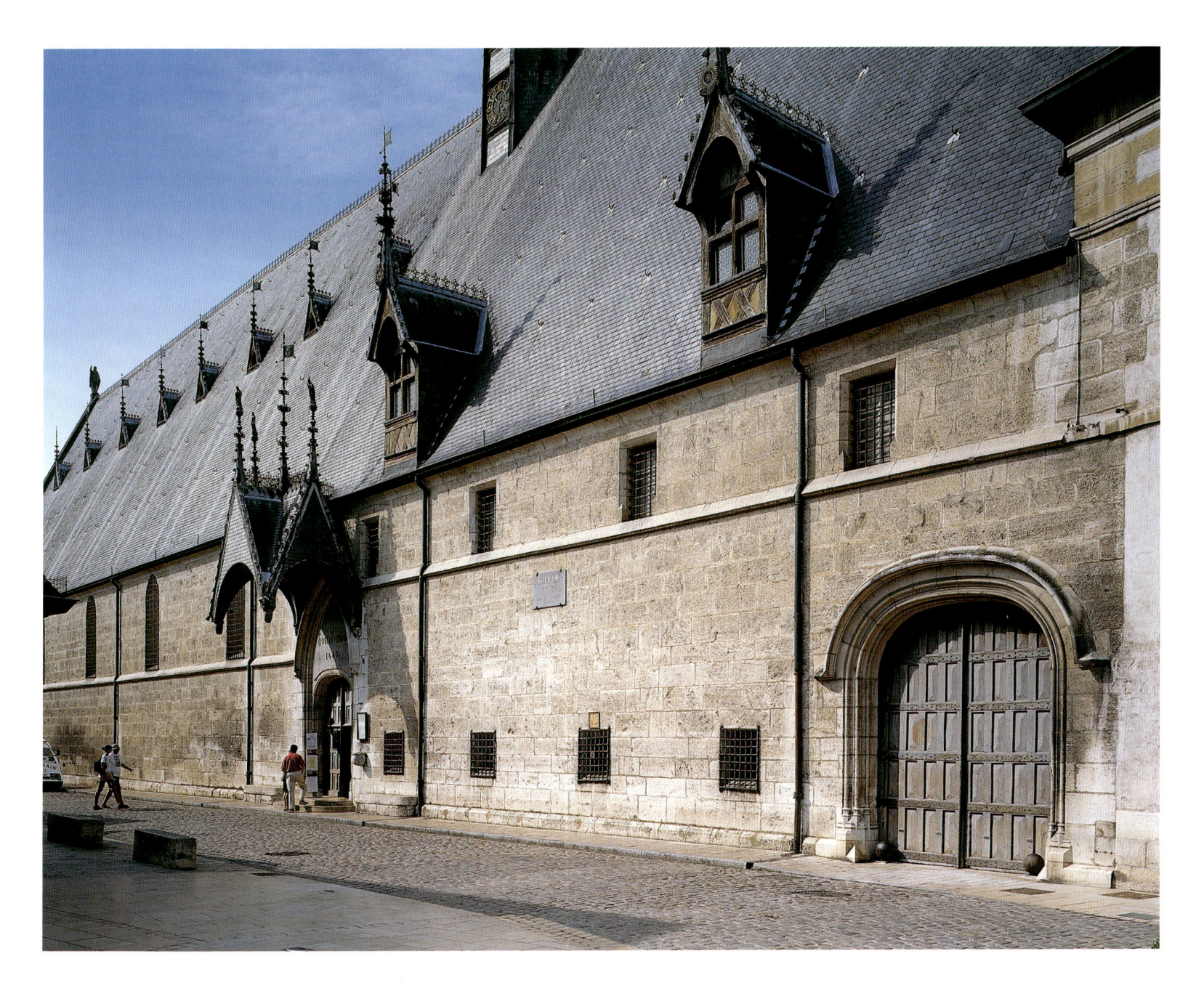

unknown architect was employed full-time by Nicolas Rolin who, like the other great *seigneurs* of his time, was constantly building, especially in his numerous residences. One thing we can be sure of, however, is that the actual work was carried out under master mason Jehan Ratheau, following a system historians have shown to be very frequent in the 15th century: the architect did not actively supervise the works, but simply made visits at intervals to assure himself that all was going according to plan.

The design of the Hôtel-Dieu was based on requirements outlined in general terms in the charter. Its focal point was the Great Hall of the Poor, set in a building looking onto the street and opposite the covered market. Entering via the vestibule, the sick were taken directly to the Great Hall by the duty sister. A smaller room, the "infirmary", awaited the "seriously ill" – those in danger of death. It was situated far from the street at the junction of the two wings forming an L-shape around the courtyard.

▌Above: The Hôtel-Dieu seen from the street.

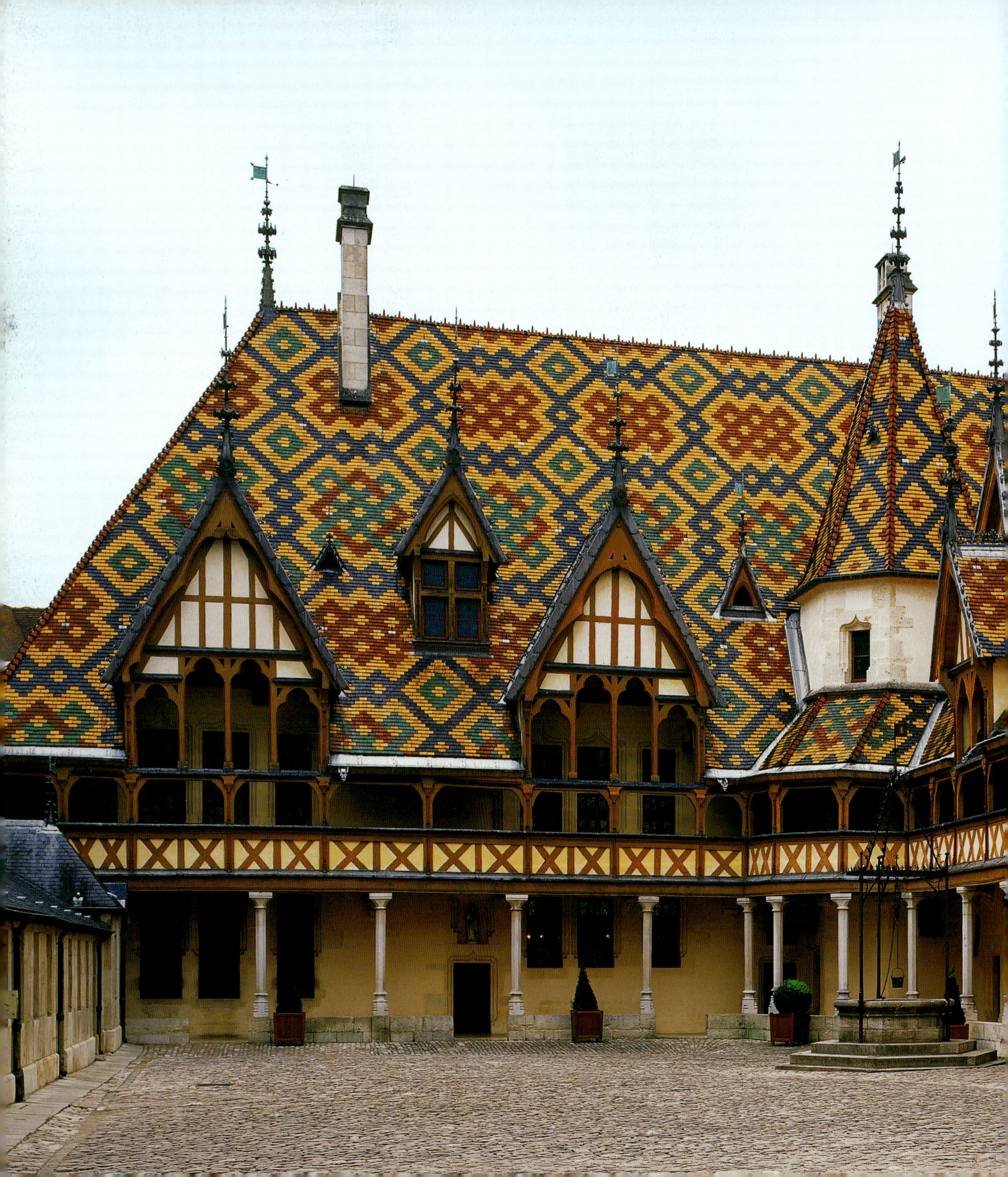

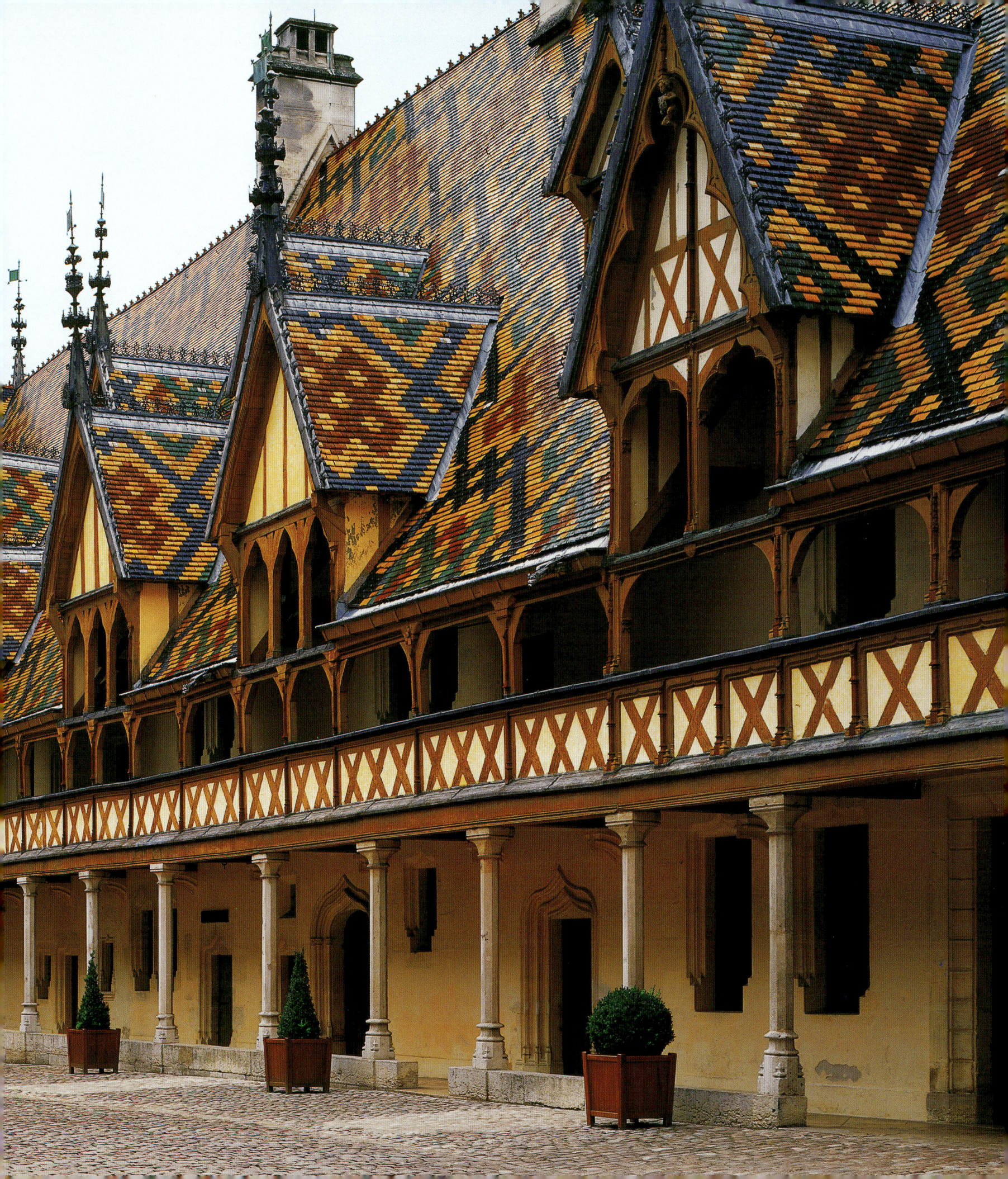

On the ground and first floor of these wings were the utility rooms and private accommodation. For the staff to be able to move about without being exposed to the elements, especially when ferrying meals, galleries ran along the courtyard side of each wing; and since the needs of the hospital meant these galleries had to be wider than those of private homes, they prevented a great deal of light from reaching the upstairs rooms. Counter-measures were taken in the form of large gabled dormer windows set into the roof above the windows of each room.

However, any proper grasp of the plan of the building calls for an understanding of an essential feature of the project: water.

WATER

A hospital of this size needed abundant supplies of running water, both for the flushing away of waste and the sheer quantity of laundry. When Nicolas Rolin went looking for a site for his hospital, the deciding factor was the offer of land traversed by the river Bouzaise. In 1442 he set about acquiring the area bounded by the covered market, the Franciscan monastery, the city wall and the street of the fishmongers. The plan of the building was determined by the course of the river, which ran all the way along the back of the allotment. With two thirds of its length along the river, the large wing at the far end of the courtyard would contain all the utility rooms and the laundry; the outdoor wash-house was set in the west corner of the courtyard – opposite today's pharmacy – at a point where the Bouzaise still flowed in the open air. It was here, in the 17th century, that sister Marie Chapon fell in and was almost drowned as she was emptying the patients' bedpans.

Before the large courtyard wing could be built the river had to be diverted and covered over. In April 1448 carts brought the "nine arches for vaulting the river", to be installed by the carpenters. Wells provided water for drinking, cooking, washing and dishwashing: one in the courtyard right next to the kitchen and the ovens, and two others in the courtyard and the cellar, handy to the nuns' refectory. Costly and time-consuming, this business of ensuring an adequate water supply may account for the delay in finishing the project, but it demonstrates the same emphasis on efficiency as does the choice of building materials.

STONE

Cut stone being impressive but expensive, its use was restricted to the main building facing the covered market. Stark and austere, it was also intended as a reminder that this was a place where the sick, in their pain and distress, entrusted themselves to God's care. The decision to use only stone was most likely the

▌ Previous pages:
The courtyard wings.
Facing page: The upper gallery of the large courtyard wing.

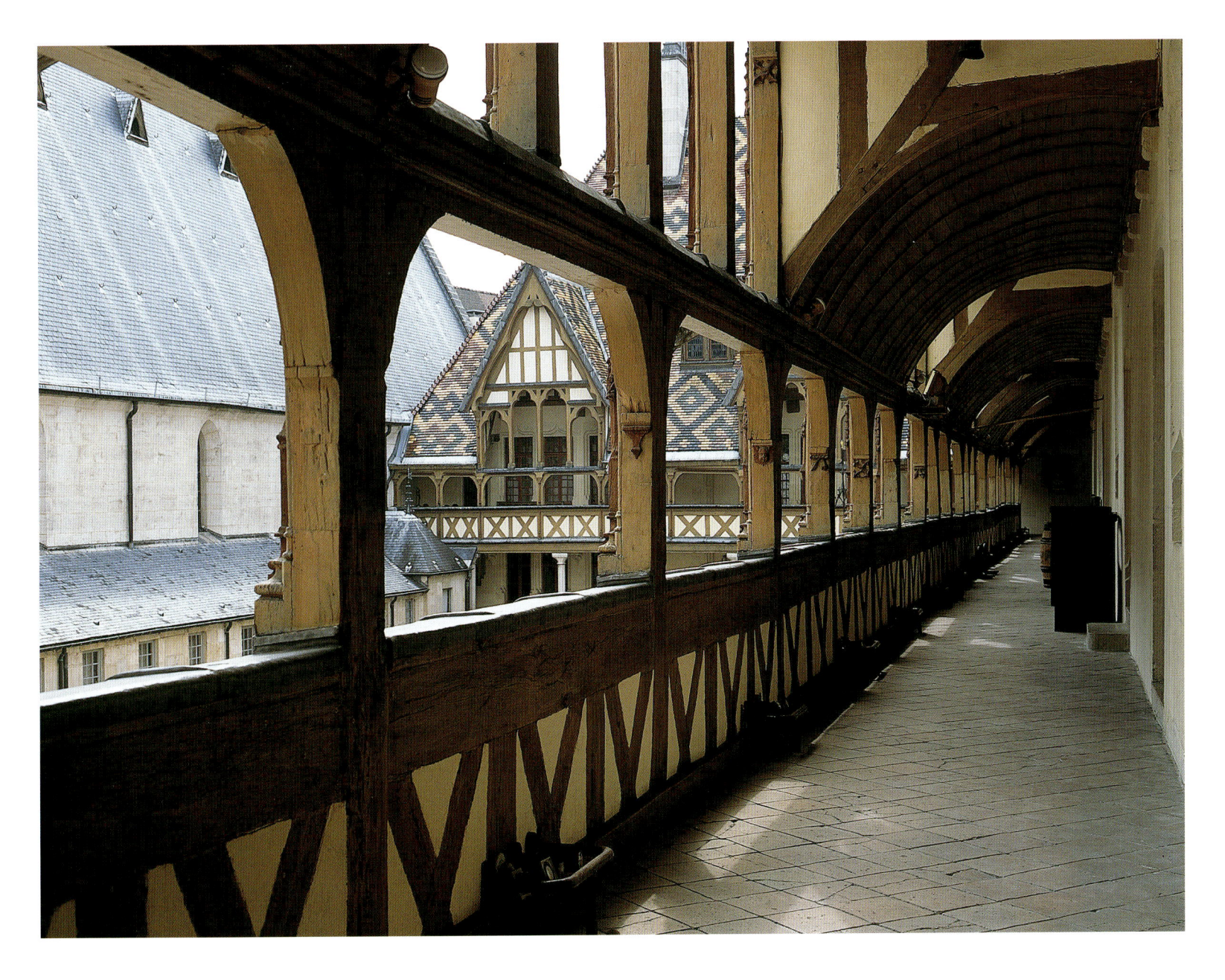

result of the fear of fire, for in 1401 Beaune had experienced a major blaze fed by the wood of the buildings inside the city walls. We know that as early as the 14th century a city like Brussels, in the heart of the Burgundian Netherlands, had taken steps to encourage the use of stone; and by 1448 facades including wood were prohibited there. It would seem that this was why, initially, there were no eaves above the entry to the Hôtel-Dieu; only a sloping porch roof that was both ugly and too close to the left-hand window of the nun's dormitory. In practical terms this was a real shortcoming, as there had to be adequate shelter for the poor who flocked to the door at eight in the morning for the "daily alms of white bread" provided by Nicolas Rolin. Ultimately the plan was altered and a double saddleback roof covered with slate and lead was created to protect the entry, whose tympanum was carved with an image of the Holy Trinity. The carving was destroyed in 1794. The facade's only decorative features were on the roof: a weathervane and lead statues of the Virgin, St John the Baptist and St Nicholas.

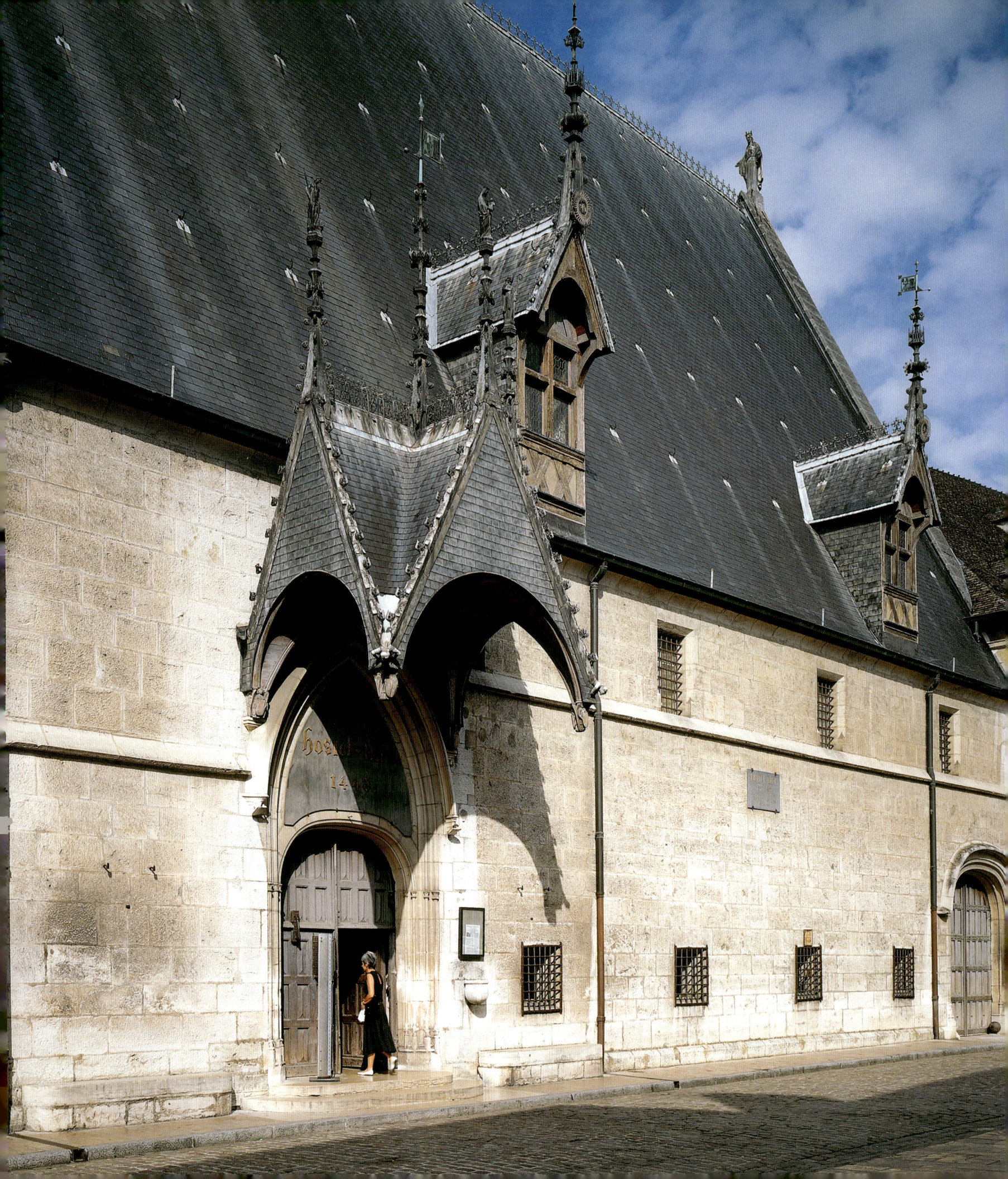

The absence of any records earlier than 1447 means we know nothing of the way the main building was constructed; but looking at the facade we can easily imagine the scaffolding the masons would have used in mounting walls slightly over a metre thick. The putlog holes – into which the carpenters inserted the pieces of wood designed to bear the scaffolding platforms – are still visible, perfectly square and spread over four levels. Some of them were filled in 1469, as pigeons had begun nesting in them.

The visitor who continues on into the courtyard is immediately struck by the contrast between the sternness of the cut stone facade and the relative exuberance of the two rear wings, with their diversity of materials and colours. Surviving account-books throw some light on the early stages of the wings, revealing that the cut stone came from the nearby quarries of Rochetain and Cochereau, the latter also being a source of rubble. However, the fifty steps for the two external spiral staircases serving the wings were ordered from Mathieu Gauchot and Pierre Garnier, who would bring them from the "stoneyard" at Blagny-sur-Vingeanne, some seventy kilometres away.

WOOD

Cut from the Duke's own forests, and in particular the "great forest of Argilly", timber arrived on the site in enormous quantities in 1447 for the rafter and truss roof of the main building. Four carpenters had made a joint bid for the contract, which was signed on 9 October 1446. Once again, lack of documentation means nothing is known of the prior carpentry work, but we can be certain that piles had to be sunk into the sodden ground, followed by the setting-up of the scaffolding and the lifting devices. The contracts and accounts relating to the roof structures of the two wings have not come down to us either, but fortunately the latter are still in their original state, apart from the sections repaired after a fire in the roof space of the large wing in 1499. Moreover, they have much to teach us, as dendrochronological analyses – tree-ring studies – have made clear.

Dendrochronology

Derived from the Greek *dendron* ("tree"), *chronos* ("time") and *logos* ("science"), dendrochronology – or tree ring analysis – is an analysis of tree growth that enables, among other things, the dating of such wood-based items as building frames, panelling, furniture and works of art. Dendrochronology can only be applied to those species of trees whose production of wood varies markedly according to climatic conditions. Oak – the favourite building wood in the Middle Ages – forms a growth ring between early spring and late summer, and if growth conditions are limiting this produces a chronological reference: less wood is produced and as a result the growth ring is narrower. In addition, oaks that have grown in similar contexts over the same period develop a series of rings with similar characteristics. This is the underlying principle of dendrochronology, with comparison indicating synchrony between series of rings and proving that they are contemporaneous.

Study of the last growth ring created during the life of a tree – the ring immediately beneath the bark – provides a dendrochronological dating that fits exactly with the year of felling. Felling may, of course, have happened at different times of the year, as was the case with the oaks used for the roof structures at the Hôtel-Dieu in Beaune.

▌Facing page: The double saddleback roof over the entrance. To the right are the windows of the nuns' dormitory and the refectory cellar.

From the forests at Argilly, Borne, Champ-Jarley and Épenôt to the roof structures of the Hôtel-Dieu

The roof structure of the main building

According to the contract of 9 October 1446 between Chancellor Nicolas Rolin and the four Beaune carpenters Jehannin Serreau, Guillemin Dudet, Guillaume La Rate and Symon Bernier, the roof frames of the main building were to be completed before Easter 1448. However it would seem from studies of the wood used that work on the "Salle des Pauvres" – the Great Hall of the Poor – continued into the summer of 1448, and on the nuns' dormitory into 1449. The contract contains a certain amount of detail as to the framing needed for the roof of the patients' dormitory, together with a summary of the roofing of the nuns' dormitory and the sacristy, and the construction of the bell-tower. The roof space for the patients' and nuns' dormitories required, among other things, more than three hundred oak trunks 14 to 16 metres long, taken from trees 30 to 37 centimetres in diameter and between 120 and 170 years old. These were chosen from the Duke's forests at Argilly, Borne, Champ-Jarley and Épenôt.

Dendrochronological studies have also shown that these enormous oaks – used for the rafters, struts and ties – were all felled during the autumn-winter of 1446-47, after the signing of the contract. After drying for several months in the forest they were carted anything from 10 to 25 kilometres to the Hôtel-Dieu site to be "squared and made ready" by the carpenters. The account books mention delivery of at least "198 rafters, 93 ties and 54 miscellaneous timbers and wallplates" over the period 27 June–14 November 1447. Smaller frame components and such secondary elements as angle braces and struts were taken from younger oaks – 80 to 100 years old – of 23-29 centimetres in diameter. While clearly from the same forests, these smaller trees were cut later, at various times between autumn/winter 1447-48 and summer 1449. Providing the wood needed to complete the frame of the main building, they were delivered, according to the account books, from January 1448 through 1450.

Even though there are gaps in the accounts, they are full of information on the advancement of the works and indicate that the summer of 1448 was a very busy period. Tree-ring analysis, in addition to pinpointing the year and season of felling, provides other details of the way things were progressing. All the indications are that the structure for the panelled roof of the patients' dormitory was in place by late July/early August 1448, a few months after Easter. This was followed by the actual lining, for which the last deliveries of panels and structural pieces had to be made before the feast of St John

■ Facing page: The roof structure of the Great Hall of the Poor.

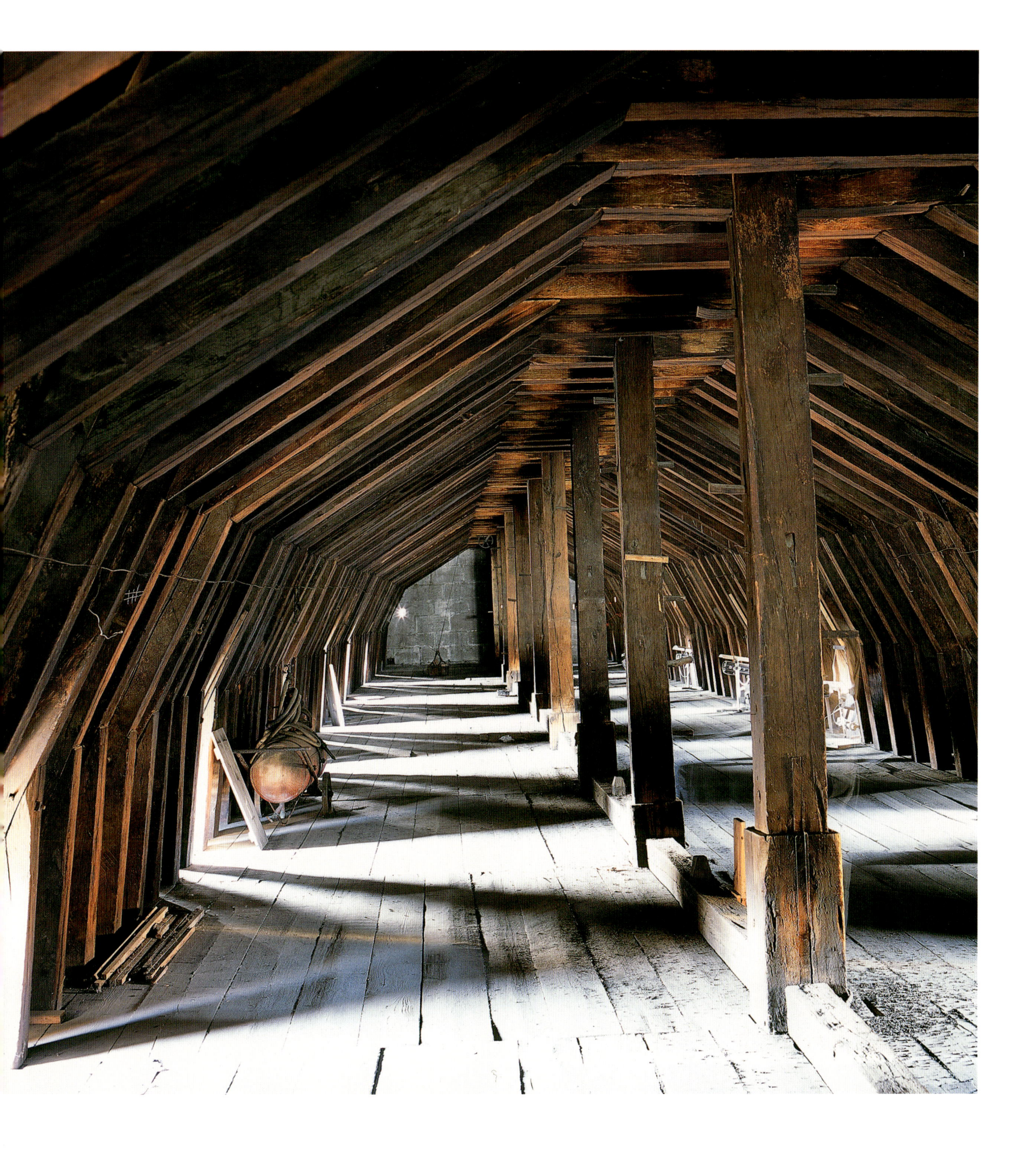

■ Above: The roof structure of the main courtyard wing.

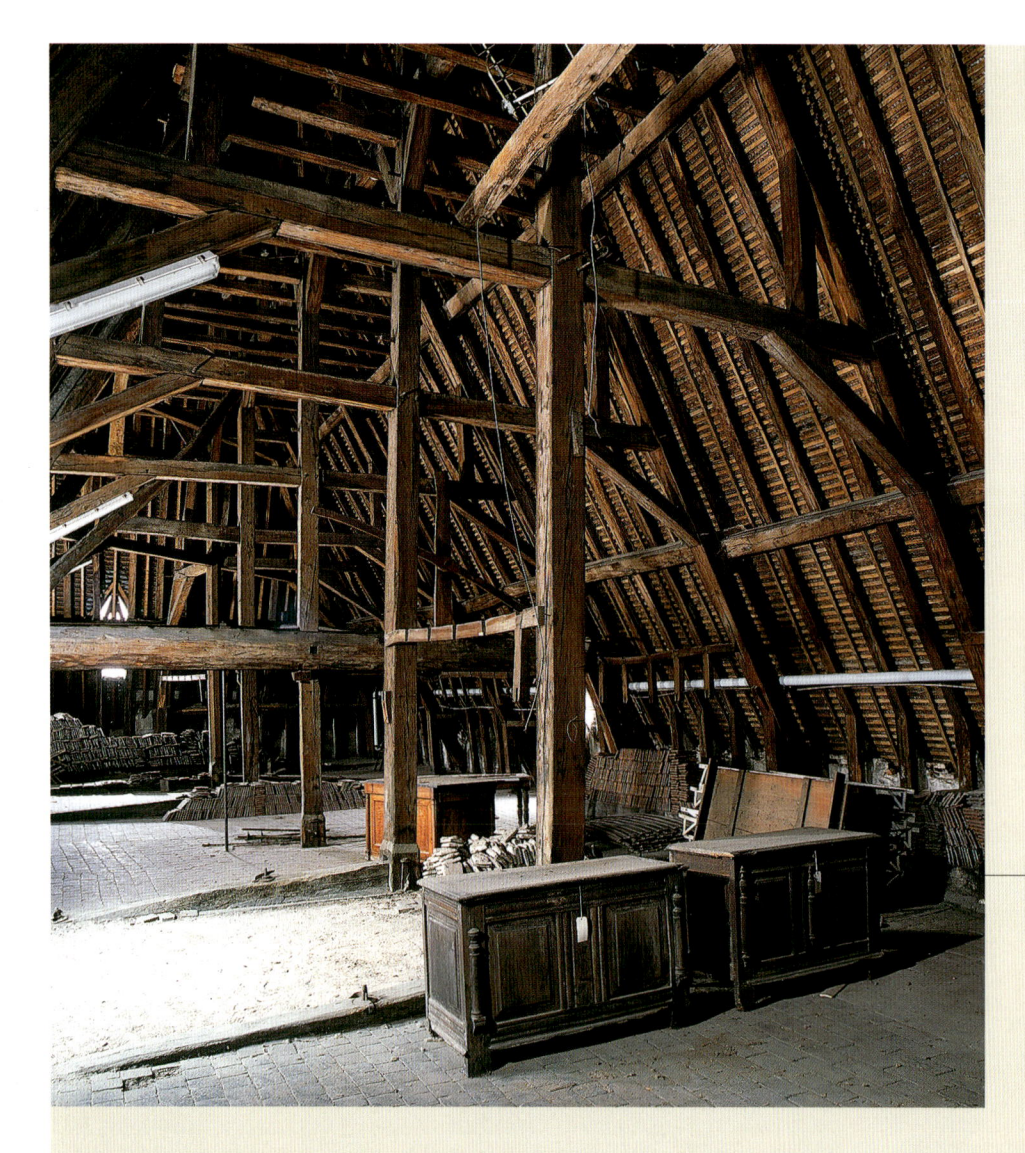

the Baptist on 24 September. For reasons that escape us, the roof frame for the nuns' dormitory, next-door to that of the patients, could not be completed at the same time, despite the express stipulation made in the contract. The necessary quantity of rafters and large carpentry pieces had certainly been available since 1447 – the final delivery of large tree trunks dated from November of that year – but the final loads of smaller wood could only have arrived after the summer of 1448, the last dendrochrono-logically identified felling period. In medieval times the cutting of trees during the spring/summer growth period – highly incompatible with successful drying and preservation – was extremely rare and usually points to such emergencies as the need to rebuild after a fire. Thus the use of oak cut during the summer of 1449 is clear evidence of a determination to get the roof space of the nuns' dormitory finished as quickly as possible.

The rear wing roof structures

The roof structures of the large and small wings on the courtyard were designed and built to a typologically unique model. They were, however, partially destroyed by fire in early 1499, the only surviving sections being those of the attics of the Chambre-Dieu and the wards known as the Salle Saint-Hugues and Salle Saint-Nicolas. These are double roofs, their interior volumes being enclosed by the principal trusses bearing longitudinal purlins which in turn carry the small rafters for the roof covering.

The main elements, such as the principal rafters, braces and ties, were taken from 120 to 160-year-old oaks of 35-42 centimetres in diameter. The smaller pieces came from younger trees – 60 to 100 years old – whose diameter rarely exceeded 30 centimetres. Studies have shown that all these trees were cut during the same period: the autumn/winter of 1449-50. In other words, the wood was available to the carpenters from then on. Once the trees had been collected and transported to the site, the squaring-off and cutting of the joints effected, and the carpentry pieces marked up, the roof structures could actually be raised, beginning most likely with that of the attic of the Chambre-Dieu. No document relating to the Hôtel-Dieu project at this time seems to have survived, but the dendrochronology indicates, in addition to the information given above, that all the oaks cut between 1446 and 1450 came from the same forests.

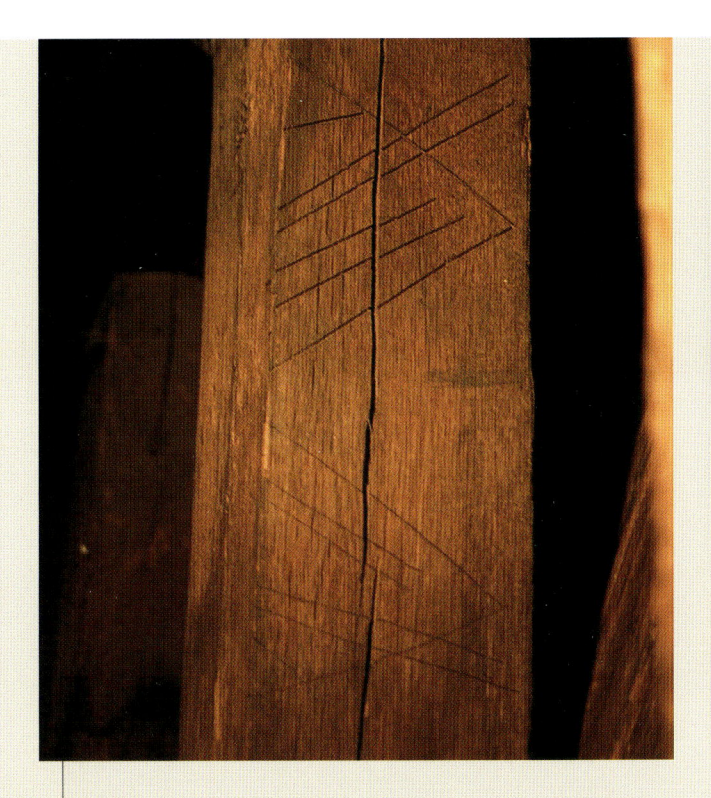

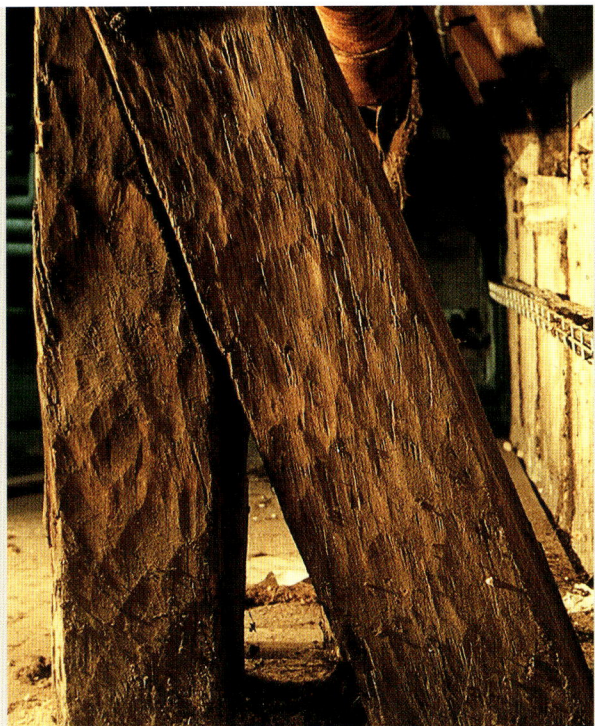

Marking up the timbers

After the felling, squaring off and sawing to length, an important stage in preparing the assembly of the roof structure was the marking up. This involved placing a mark near the assembly points of each member, a kind of reference number making for ready identification and thus helping to ensure that there were no hitches in the actual raising of the roof. In most cases Roman numerals were used, but with modifications intended to avoid any possibility of confusion in the handling of the members. For example, 4 was written IIII, to differentiate it clearly from 6, written VI or IV. Lastly, the addition of a small line, or carpenter's mark, indicated whether a given member should go to the left or the right of the axis of the truss. It was on the member's marked-up side, called the setting-out face, that the pegs were driven in; and logically it was this side that the carpenters would be looking at when the trusses were raised.

Acquaintance with the marking up process is essential to an understanding of the assembly plan and recognition of any modifications or restoration that may have ensued. The marking up of the hundreds of trusses making up the roof structure of the main wing is thoroughly consistent and possesses a distinctive feature in the survival of the preliminary marks, made with a scriber prior to the definitive marking up with a tracing iron. Most of the members also bear very clear setting-out and framing lines, as well as handsome traces left by the broadaxes and adzes used for squaring off and smoothing the surface of the wood.

▐ Left: The roof structure of the Great Hall of the Poor: detail of the preliminary marks and the definitive marking up of side post no. 27.
Right: The roof structure of the main wing on the courtyard: marks left by an adze on a side post and strut.

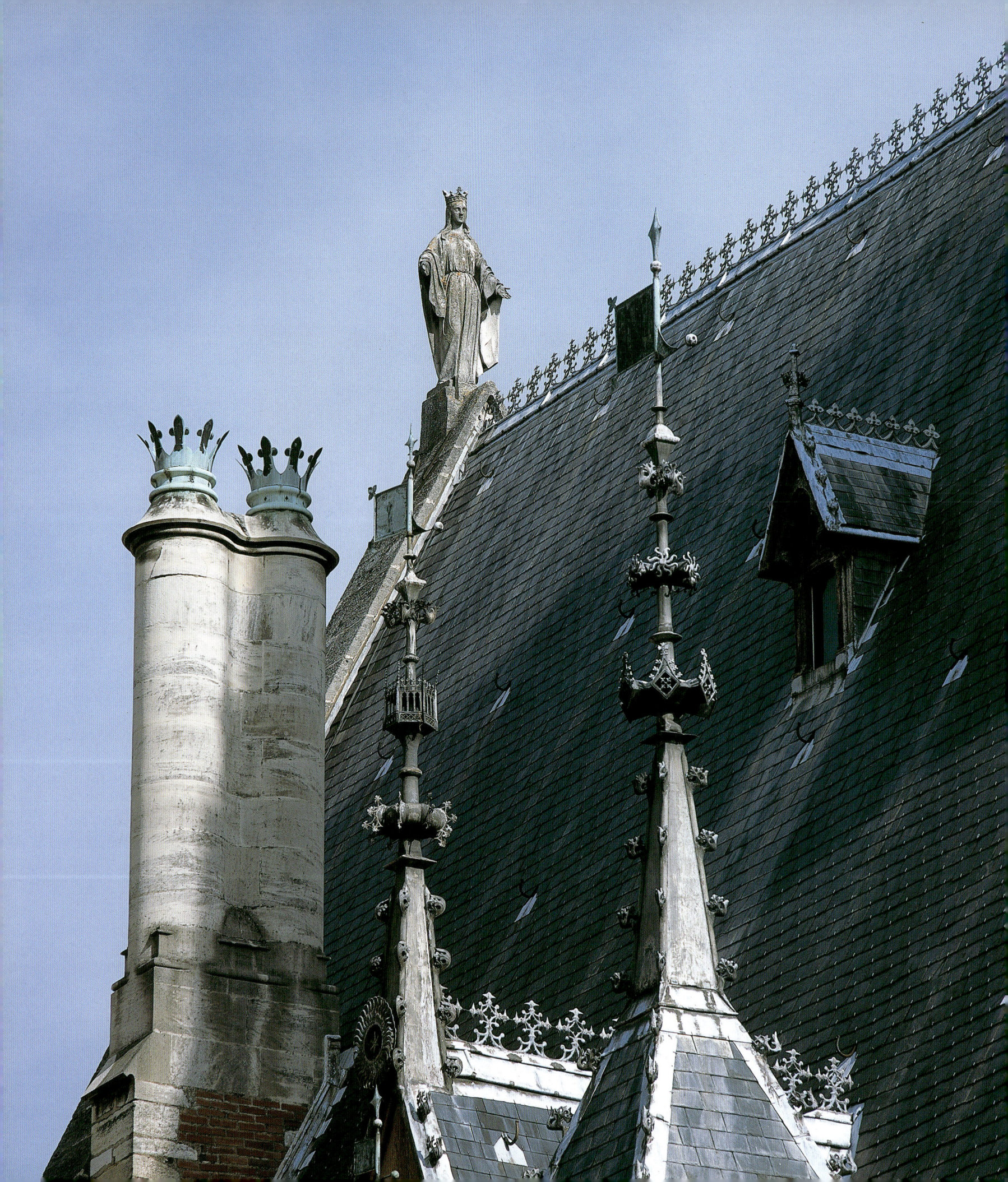

SLATE

Late in 1447 wagons from Chatenoy-le-Royal, near Chalon-sur-Saône, delivered the ten thousand slates that would be nailed and overlapped one by one on the roof of the streetside building and the belltower. Most probably despatched by river, they were doubtless from the great slate quarries at Fumay and Rimogne, near Charleville-Mézières in the distant Ardennes. It was from Charleville-Mézières, too, that the roof-tiler Baudechon Courtois would come. An expensive item — all the more so because it came from so far away — slate was ideal for steeply sloping roofs: now tiled, the dovecote and the staircase turrets were originally covered with slate.

CLAY

In spite of the wealth of clay in Burgundy, roof and paving tiles remained expensive. What was doubtless the first load of tiles was delivered in 1448, destined for the "vestry", the sacristy built onto the gable wall on the Franciscan monastery side. These were ordinary tiles, as opposed to the more durable "leaded" type, so called because of their protective coat of lead glaze. The composition of the glaze could be varied to produce a range of colours that made possible the polychrome, geometrically patterned roofs found in Burgundy and elsewhere. Nothing is known of the tiles ordered for the two rear wings, but they were certainly lead-glazed.

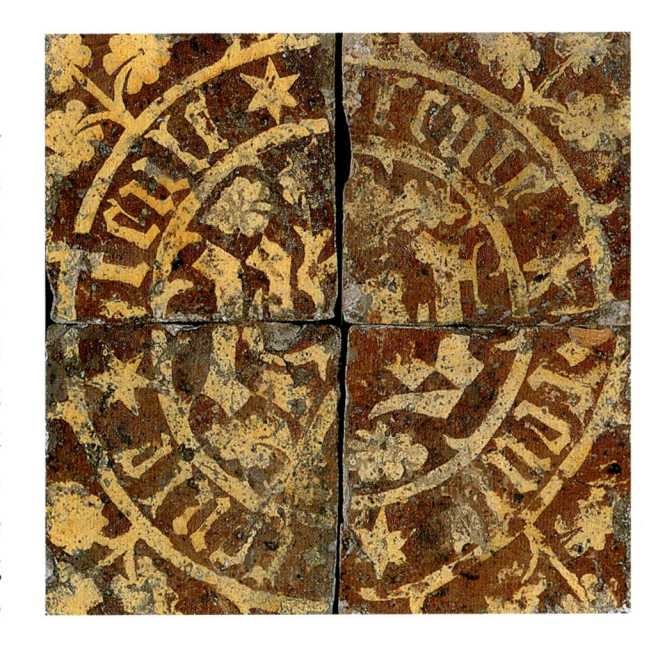

Curiously, there is no allusion in the archives to polychrome tiles and no early description of them; the only evidence is a straw model of the building dating from the mid-18th century. The flamboyantly coloured roofs so admired by visitors today — they have become the very symbol of the Hôtel-Dieu in Beaune — were reinvented as the 20th century got under way by Sauvageot, an architect from the Department of Historical Monuments. His starting point was the straw model, a handful of old tiles suggesting different colours, and a section of roof then covered with "glazed tiles forming a glossy, multicoloured, geometrical design." As it happened

▮ Facing page: The roof of the main streetside building; statue of the Virgin Mary sculpted by Étienne de Saptes in the 19th century. Above: 15th-century paving tiles bearing Nicolas Rolin's motto and the initials N.G., associating the founder's first name with that of his wife, Guigone de Salins.

this area of roof was not ancient at all, having been – as a contemporary postcard testifies – an exercise in restoration undertaken in 1883 by the Hospices de Beaune architect Félix Goin, working from a drawing by Maurice Ouradou. In the course of the work carried out under Sauvageot in 1902-07, the roofers found tiles bearing what might be the stamp of Jehan Digart, who had made them in 1448.

It is likely that most of the floor areas were paved with terracotta tiles – glazed or unglazed, plain or decorated. The 1448 accounts reveal a delivery of 6000 plain, unglazed tiles and an order for 50,000 lead-glazed ones whose slip decoration was to be Nicolas Rolin's "livery" as already used in his Dijon townhouse. The "livery" was basically the initials NG and the motto "Alone" – adopted by Rolin at the time of his third marriage to Guigone de Salins in 1423 – followed by a star. The overall design comprised four tiles and was stamped into the unfired clay with four wooden matrices made by the Dijon image cutter Jehannin Fouquerel. These four tiles, "with their proportions slightly enlarged", were used as a model in the 1870s, when the Boch Brothers company made stoneware paving for the floors of a number of rooms.

An independent – i.e. non-ducal – tilery run by Denisot Jeot at Aubigny-en-Plaine manufactured the 50,000 tiles delivered in 1448, of which 8200 were undecorated: as a rule these latter were used to edge and frame the decorated tiles. It has been calculated that the 50,000 tiles would pave 911 square metres: the Great Hall of the Poor alone accounted for 619 square metres.

METAL

Generally speaking, large-scale medieval building projects had their own on-site forge for making the necessary ironwork. This did not, however, exclude the purchase of such readymade items as fastening components, nails, grilles, hinges, locks, door furniture and tools. In 1447-1448 Jehan Champenois delivered large quantities of muck-iron and hammered iron – latticework, strips, frames – together with 64,000 nails. The two pieces of ironwork that give such character to the main door were replaced with exact copies in 1882-83: a "one-quarter scale" drawing by Maurice Ouradou shows the grille of the spyhole and the strange knocker that seems to portray a slowworm about to gulp down a fly.

While large quantities of lead went into securing window panes and stained glass, preparing glaze for the paving tiles and perhaps making water pipes, for the most part it was used for the various roof ornaments: crests, finials, suns, roses, crowns, and plant and architectural motifs, some of which were designed to prevent leaks. These ornaments were then painted, gilded or tinned. In Poland, where lead was plentiful, this kind of roof ornamentation had

■ Facing page: The knocker and spyhole grille at the entrance: these are identical late 19th-century copies of the originals.

made its appearance in the 14th century. In 1702 the board of directors decided not to replace the decor around the base of the belltower: a lot of money had already been spent and it was felt that there was no real need for the embellishments described in 1653 by one J. Grozelier as "the coats of arms and escutcheons, painted on lead, of the houses of Vienne, Vergy, Châlon, Luxembourg and others I could not identify, the aforementioned blazons and arms having been partly effaced by the assaults of time." The missing items were replaced in 1843. The roofs also bore numerous weathervanes – a privilege restricted to the nobility – in the form of banners painted with Nicolas Rolin's coat of arms: "Azure three keys or paleways". Over the years all these decorative pieces have been restored several times. While the building of the Hôtel-Dieu has a frankly ostentatious side in terms both of design and choice of materials, it must be admitted that there was also an underlying concern with quality and solidity – with the creation of something that would endure.

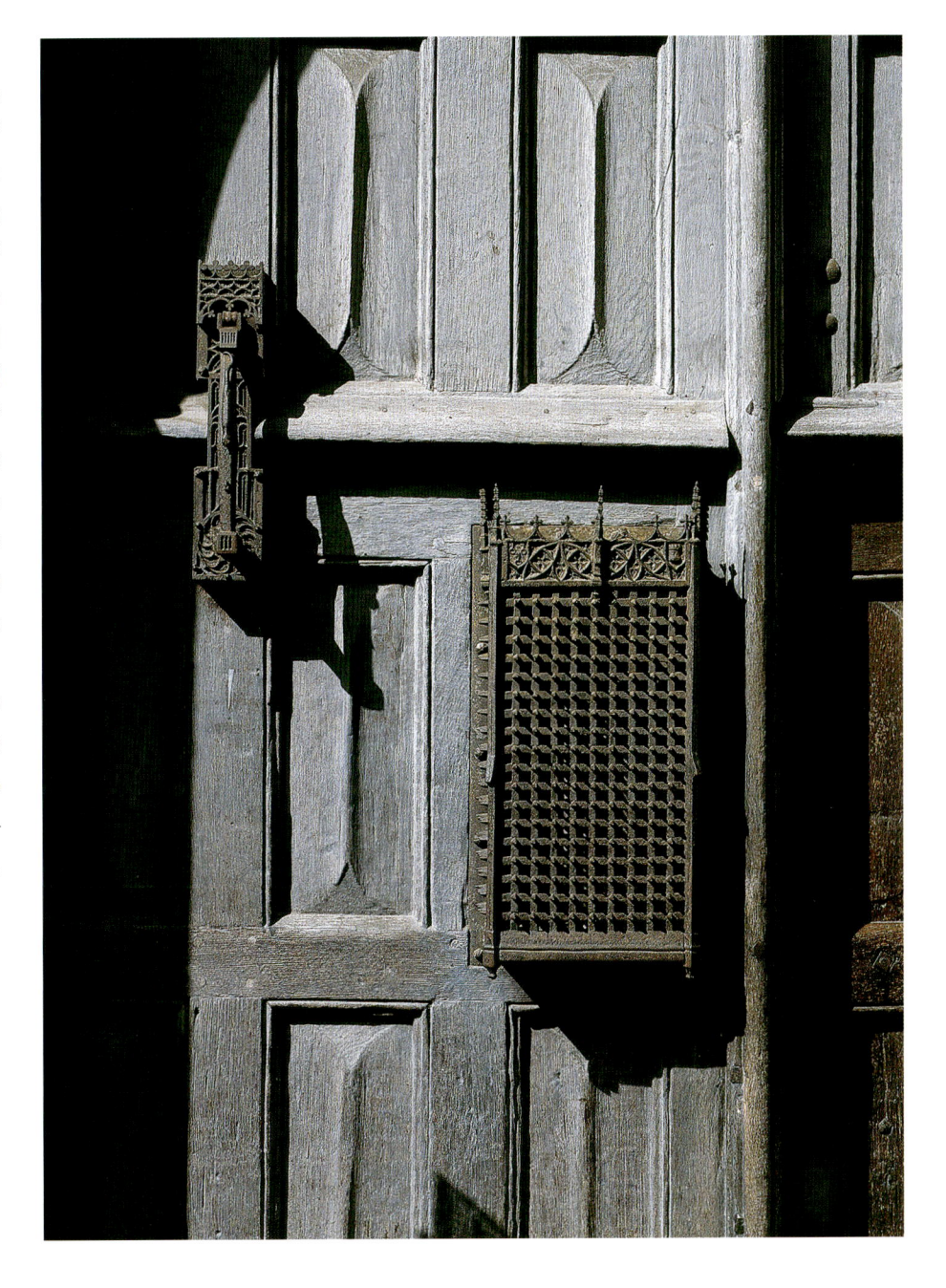

The evolution of a 15th-century building

It is because Nicolas Rolin demanded an annual list of the furnishings in the Hôtel-Dieu that we now possess a document crucial to our overall knowledge of the building: the inventory of 1501. At the beginning of the 16th century the Hôtel-Dieu had two large halls for the sick poor, eight private wards, utility rooms, a barn housing a winepress, various rooms for the nuns and "two little rooms with fireplaces for restraining the sick poor when they become agitated and take leave of their senses". These last seem to have been little used for this purpose, serving mostly as storerooms for spinning wheels and the clothing of deceased patients.

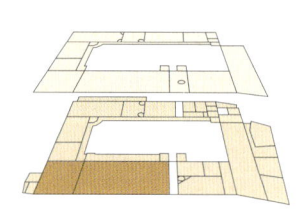

THE GREAT HALL OF THE POOR AND THE CHAPEL

In 1443 Nicolas Rolin had declared that "there will be made and laid out, in the main building and near the chapel of the aforementioned hospital, thirty beds: fifteen along one side of the aforementioned building and fifteen along the other." He was referring to the Great Hall of the Poor, overtly churchlike in size and design. It could accommodate up to sixty patients, each bed serving "for one sick person and often two". The Hall became operational on 1 January 1452.

On entering for the first time patients must have been dazzled by the furnishings, the gleam of the terracotta tiles and the profusion of colours of the paintings, stained glass and fabrics. Yet they could not but be struck by Rogier Van der Weyden's *Last Judgement* polyptych, set majestically on the high altar at the far end. Through the latticework of the high wooden partition separating off the chapel, sumptuous furniture could be glimpsed. In the nearer part of the hall were the beds with their white curtains and the cupboards in which the hospital personnel stored the pewterware and bed linen. In front of the chapel, near the lower gallery through which the nuns brought the meals, was a long table covered with a cloth, at which the patients ate when summoned by a bell hanging near the main door.

At the head of each bed was a recess in the wall for small personal items. Naturally there was no fireplace in this enormous room – 46.2 x 13.4 metres – with its panelled pointed barrel ceiling. At the time there was nothing exceptional about this type of roof, which left the middle-posts and ties visible: the combination of its considerable height and openings in the panelling meant that this wooden vault ensured good ventilation for the hall. In addition, eight pointed-arch windows set high above the beds provided ventilation without inconveniencing the patients. The nuns tried in vain to compensate for the lack of heating with hot-water bottles, warming pans and a "table heater".

With the exception of the roof structure and the cut stone walls, the Great Hall has lost some of its authenticity: its present state is the result of a Neo-Gothic

■ Facing page: The chapel.

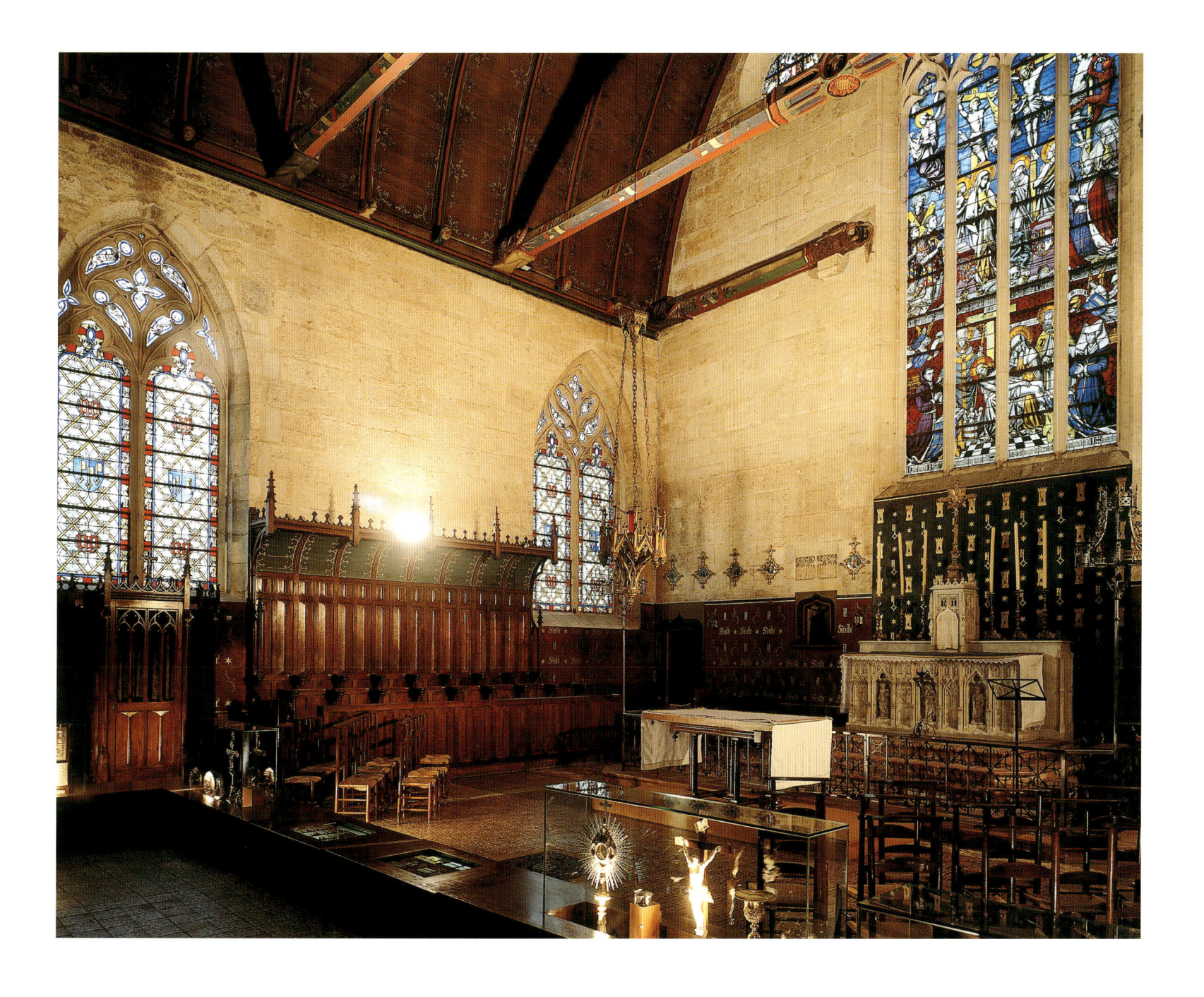

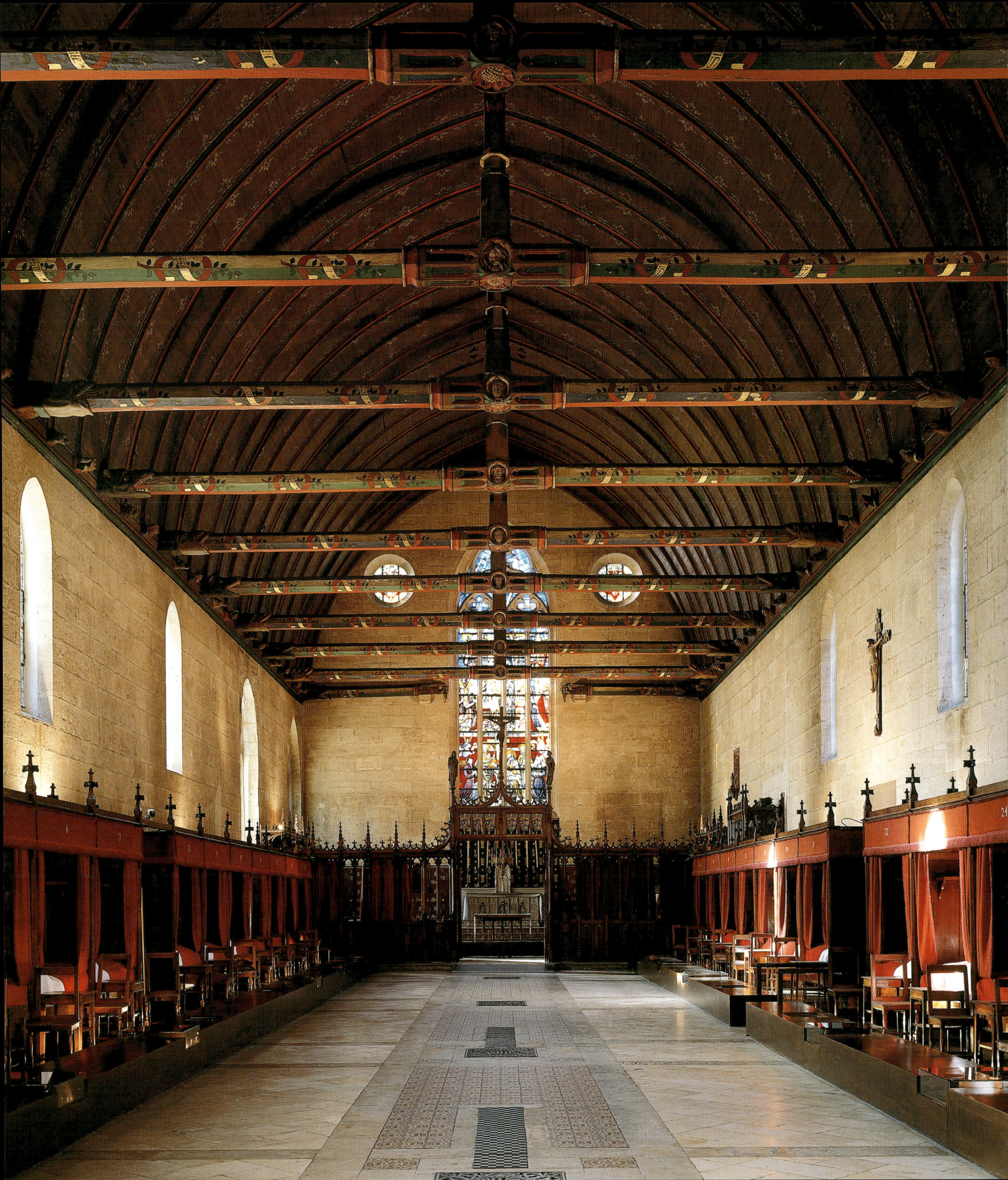

restoration undertaken in 1872-78 by Maurice Ouradou (1822-84), pupil, son-in-law and fervent admirer of Viollet-le-Duc. To be sure, time had taken its toll on the hall since the 15th century. In 1802, even though the room had been closed for two years because of its dilapidation, the administrators had discussed its possible use as a dormitory for the nuns, whose original sleeping quarters had been judged "uncomfortable and unsanitary". To this end a floor had been laid over the ties of the roof frame, but things went no further. The splendid stained glass window over the high altar had been destroyed during the Revolution and in 1802 the bay was walled off up to the height of the added floor. By 1845 it had been agreed that the hall should be restored in the 15th-century style, but architect Pierre-Paul Petit's project was disregarded. Twenty years later a specialist was called in, in the form of Maurice Ouradou, who – under the supervision of his father-in-law – had taken part in the restoration of the medieval château at Pierrefonds, north of Paris. Presented in 1872, his proposals began with "complete restoration of the great panelled vault via restoration of the paintings". The earlier décor of "paintings, foliations, emblems and coats of arms" became visible when the coat of whitewash was removed. Then, after initially serving as scaffolding, the floor created in 1802 would be removed and the walls decorated.

The project evolved in the course of the works, as Ouradou himself explained: "I am delighted to have rediscovered, under coat after coat of whitewash, most of the main elements of the overall décor; and I was greatly helped for the rest by the detailed description in an inventory dating from 1501, found in the Hôtel-Dieu archives. This inventory, of whose existence I was not aware when I drew up my project, together with the discoveries I had the good fortune to make once work had begun, obliged me to change some of my plans, notably regarding the large stained

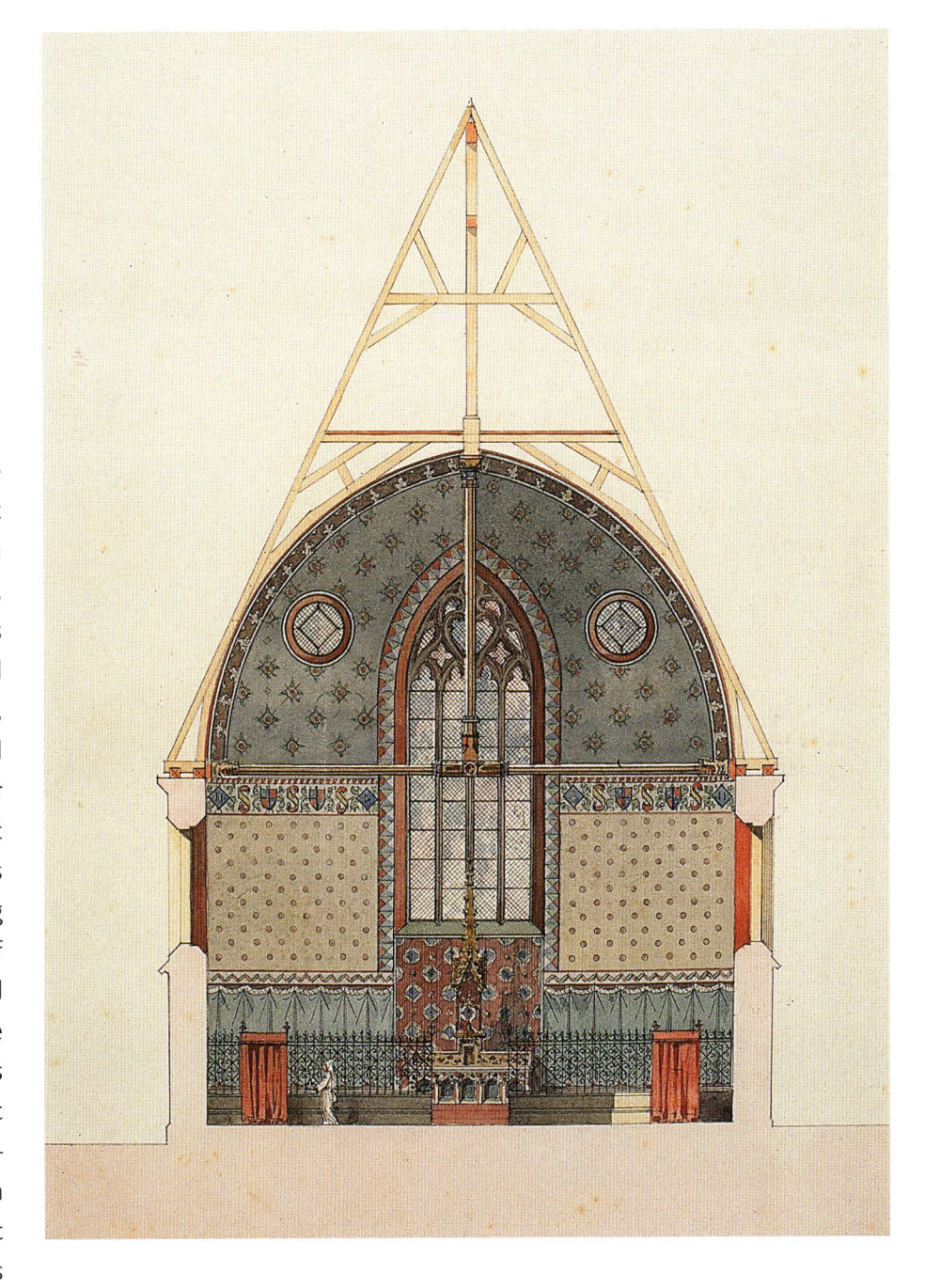

▌Facing page: The Great Hall of the Poor and its chapel.
Above: Maurice Ouradou's restoration plan for the chapel, 1872.

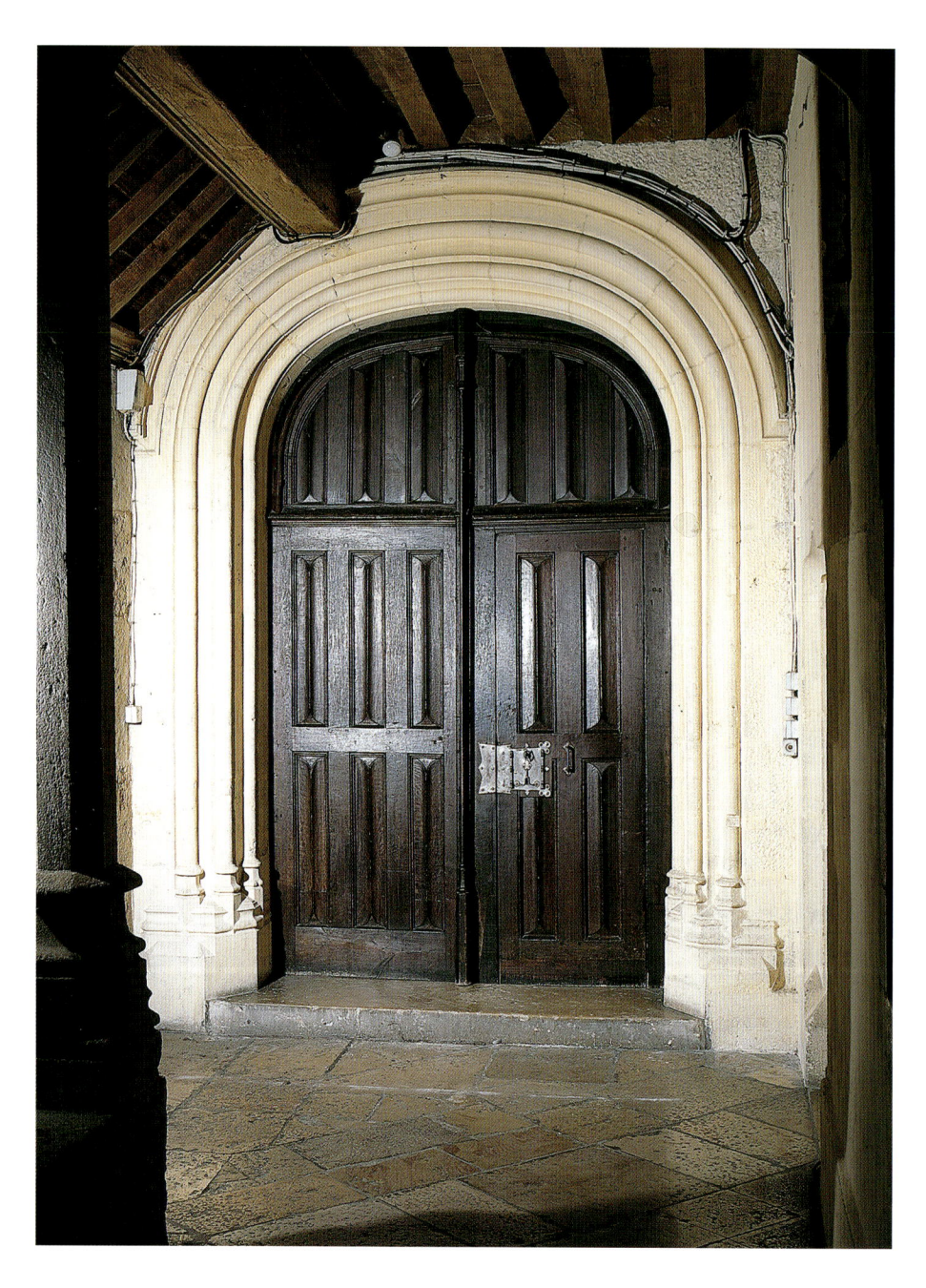

glass window, the furniture, the panelling, etc." His estimate had made provision for a wrought iron grille between the chapel and the rest of the room, but he finally opted for a panelled partition with latticework, as indicated in the 1501 inventory. However, he brought the partition forward so as to spare the patients the sight of the "funeral corteges" that now filed directly from the lower gallery into the chapel. Ouradou had demanded workmen combining "acknowledged skill, with experience of the decorative style of the Middle Ages acquired in the course of similar projects, and able to provide the necessary proof of this." The Beaune sculptor Benjamin Bernard restored the sculptures on the roof structure, damaged during the installation of the floor: this involved recreating the faces and heads on the ties and restoring all the animal heads, together with some of the human ones, on the struts. Restored by the stonemason Combre-Pommier, the great window over the high altar recovered its original function: the new stained glass pane created by Parisian master glassmaker Léon-Auguste Ottin took its inspiration from its predecessor. Pasquinelly-Bruley, from Beaune, painted new ornamentation on the ceiling panels, following full-size drawings provided by Ouradou.

Since the 1820s the walls had been covered with painted mock-marble: Ouradou replaced this, in the hall, with an imitation cut stone motif – a common approach since the 13th century – and a frieze bearing the arms of Nicolas Rolin and his wife.

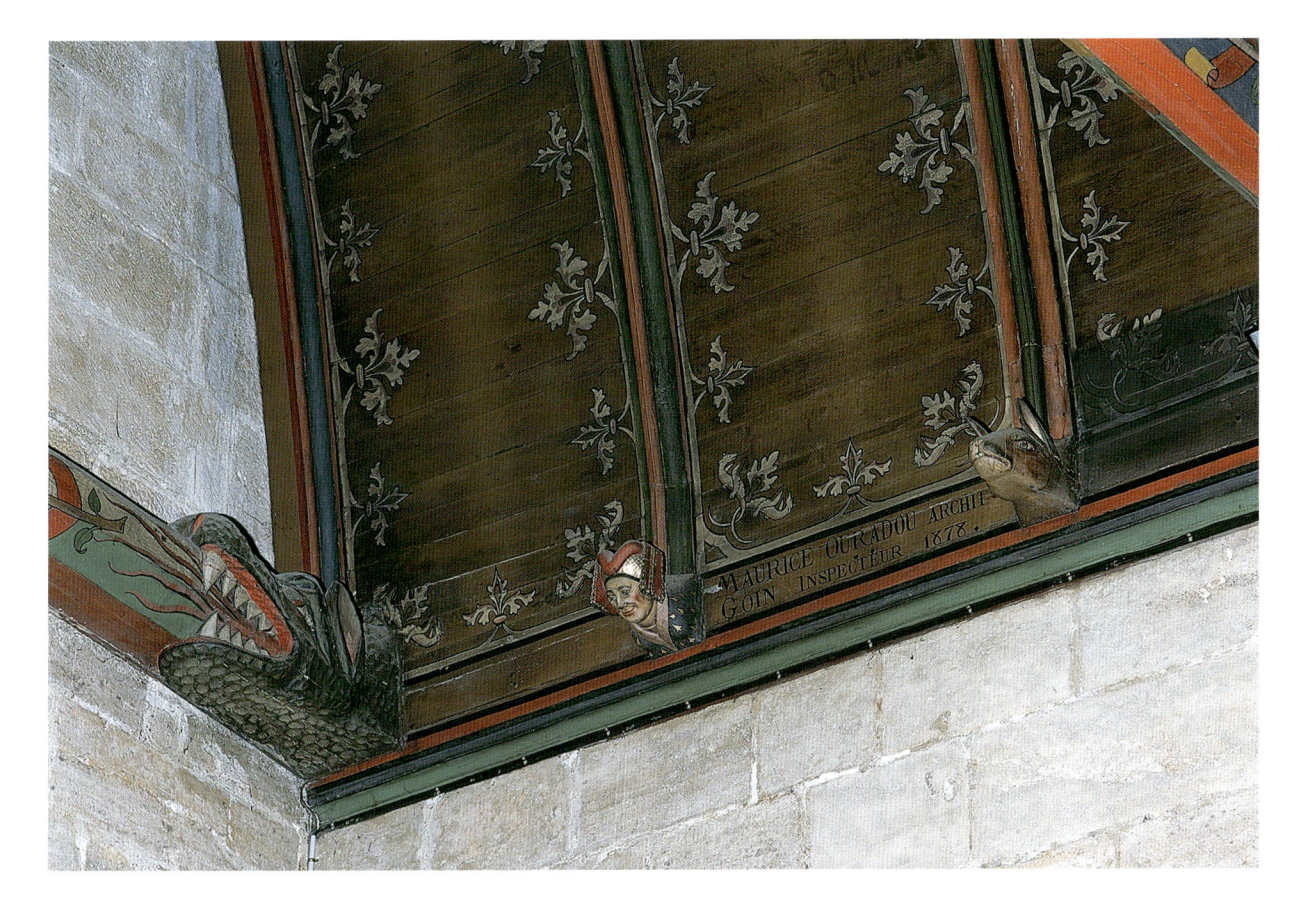

Facing page: The door to the chapel, seen from the lower gallery.
Left: Struts in the shape of a woman's head and animals' heads.

However, in the chapel he opted for a more sophisticated décor reproducing the famed tapestries – doves on a red background – contemporary with the founding of the Hôtel-Dieu. With the exception of a witness sample, the false stonework was done away with in the 20th century.

The 1872 restoration of the Great Hall gave the directors a long-awaited chance to deal with the heating problem, using a furnace and "a system specially designed for the ventilation and salubrity of such an enormous sickroom, with heat vents, footwarmers and expulsion of contaminated air." The area in front of the altar was dug out in search of the vault in which Guigone de Salins had been buried in 1470; the small tomb was found – it had been vandalised during the Revolution – and used to house the heating ducts. The restoration of the hall was rounded off with the laying of a new stone floor including a "central aisle

Facing page: The salle Saint-Nicolas: site of the medieval ovens, then of the old women's infirmary.

with coloured tiles representing a carpet". With the single exception of the white marble altar, in place since 1845, all the furnishings, including the beds, were recreated according to Ouradou's drawings. After six years' work the Great Hall began receiving patients again on 17 July 1878.

Dating from 1804, the long lean-to type building attached to the courtyard side of the Great Hall had been added "as a service area and for storage of the linen needed daily by the patients".

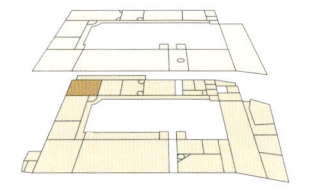

THE "INFIRMARY FOR THE GRIEVOUSLY ILL"

In 1653 this room for the dying was described as containing "thirteen beds occupied by poor, failing patients and crippled, wounded soldiers, some of them in their death agony and the others in terrible straits." They had a view of an altar set beneath a "picture telling three stories": the crucifixion, the adoration of the Magi and the flight into Egypt. To ensure a sufficient volume of air, the infirmary took up the full height of the building, with a ceiling set on exposed joists and, out of consideration for its unfortunate occupants, a fireplace. In 1659 the windows opening onto the garden were replaced with tall, arched openings; this was made possible by the generosity of Hugues Bétauld, founder of the Salle Saint-Hugues ward.

When Louis XIV visited in 1658 he asked that men and women patients be separated for reasons of propriety, but the infirmary remained mixed. A hundred years later the building of a second room for women was mooted, but the choice of a site was problematical: "With regard to the riverbed and the convenience of both patients and nuns, it was desirable that the two infirmaries should be adjoining and even communicating via doors the patients could not use, only the nuns being provided with keys." There was, then, no other solution than to demolish the "upper and lower-level rooms" occupied by the ovens, the flour store and the patients' latrines on the gallery side of the ground floor: "These facilities gave off such a stench that when there were processions special pellets had to be burned over them."

These major works were undertaken in 1754: after partial demolition of the wall between the medieval infirmary and the ovens, a large arch was cut in it to mark the separation. Placed under the arch so as to be shared by the two halls was a double-sided altar, flanked with curtained grills that prevented all movement and communication between the patients. On each side of the altar were "holes falling into the river to carry away the water from the baths and elsewhere". To meet the heating, ventilation and lighting requirements a fireplace was built backing onto the one in the kitchen and three tall arched windows, identical to those of the 17th century, were created. The "two small rooms overhanging the

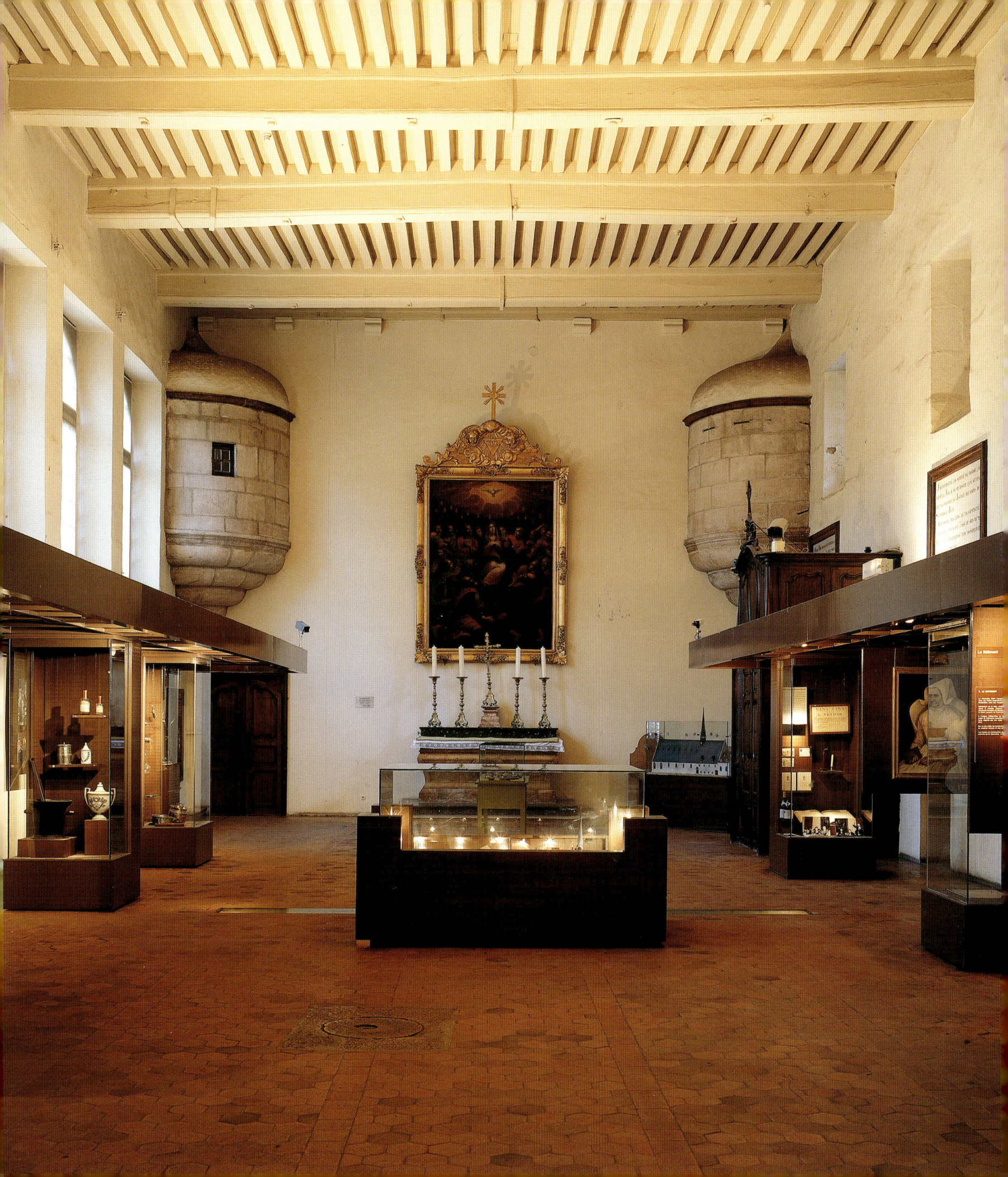

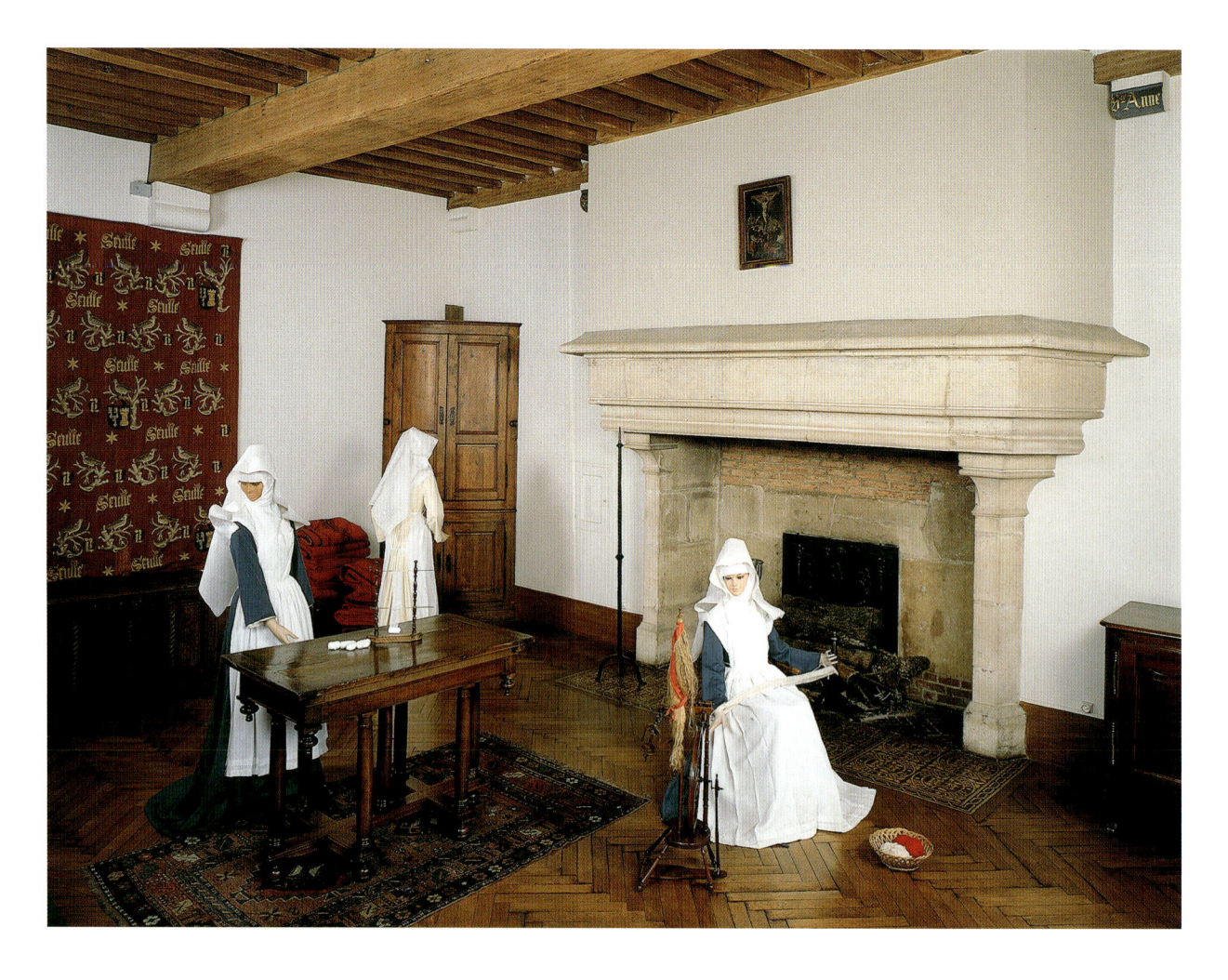

Above: The former Salle Sainte-Anne.
Facing page: The Salle Saint-Hugues.

corners of the hall on squinches" do not each have the same function: one was a surveillance post while the other housed the nuns' latrines, next-door to their infirmary. To service the new hall a diversion canal some 3.2 metres wide and 2.5 metres deep was dug to bring water from the river through the garden, "so that all the linen and utensils can be washed there and all the refuse thrown in will be carried away." A row of small adjoining outbuildings was constructed along this canal.

Major works in 1847 and then in 1867 put an end to this separate existence, the new joint infirmary being dedicated to St Nicholas in memory of the Hôtel-Dieu's founder. After continuing to receive patients until 1980, it was totally restored in 1986-87 by the architect Frédéric Didier of the Department of Historical Monuments.

THE PRIVATE ROOMS

Set in the ground and first floors of the two courtyard wings, the private rooms also changed over time. Despite their terracotta floor tiles bearing the founder's motto, exposed-joist ceilings, fireplaces and elaborate furnishings, they were not all equally well lit. The four rooms of the small wing were dark, for the only windows they had gave onto the galleries. At the request of the monks the opposite wall, on the Franciscan monastery side, had to remain windowless. Only the Salle Notre-Dame on the first floor had lay-lights in the wall separating it from the patients in danger of death. By contrast all the rooms in the large wing were lit from both the courtyard and the garden on the south side. For all these rooms the 1501 inventory lists an altar and a large bed, together with one

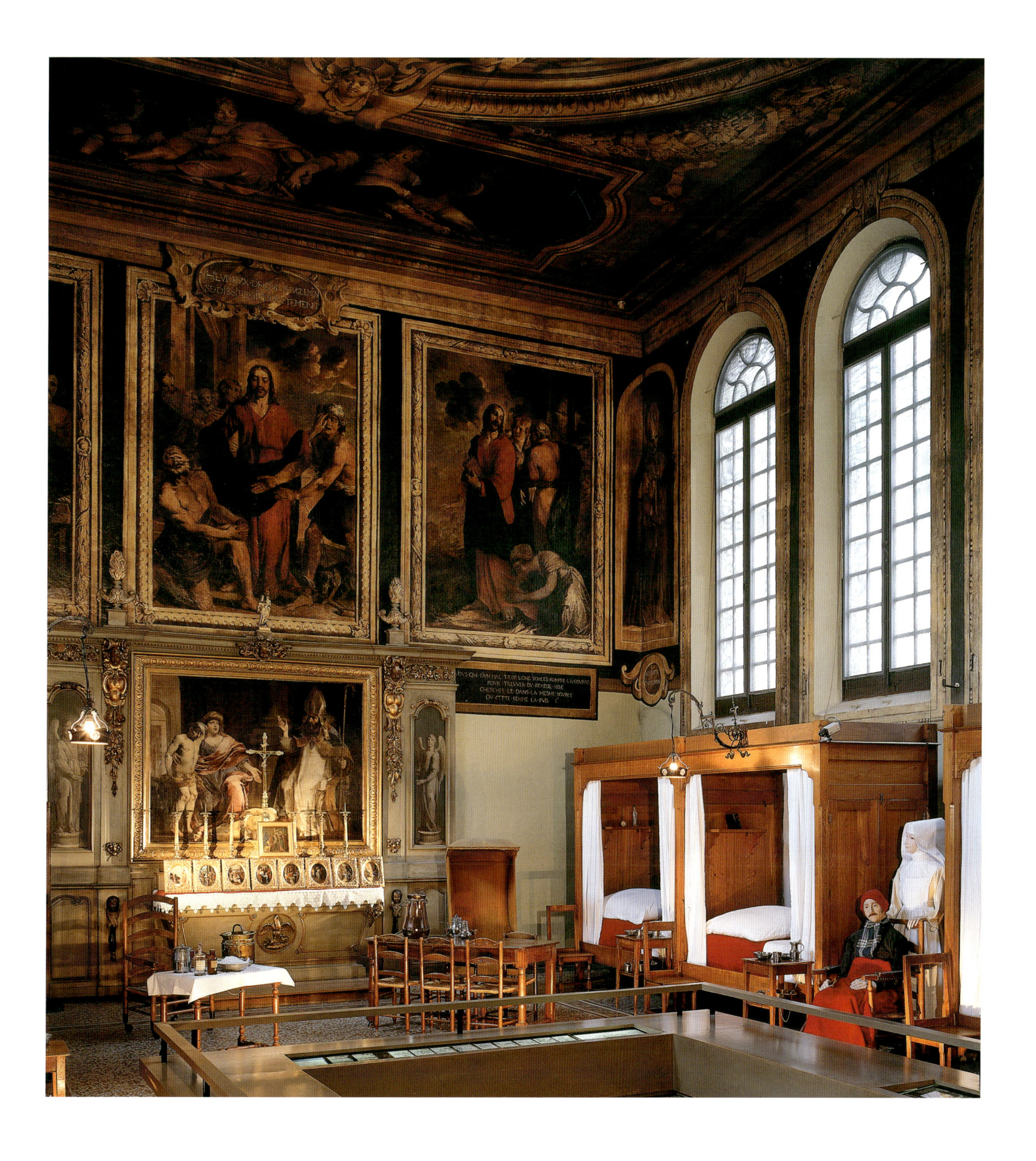

■ Below:
Virgin and Child, earthenware plate from the "little museum", Nevers, 17th century(?)
Facing page:
The boardroom, redesigned in the late 19th century.

to three additional beds. The Salle Sainte-Marthe was the only one to have six large beds; curiously it had no altar, a feature that may be explained by refurbishing subsequent to the death of Nicolas Rolin.

The Salle Sainte-Anne, next-door to the Great Hall and unique in still having its medieval fireplace, underwent major alterations in 1696 and then in 1788. In 1693 François Brunet de Montforand had made a bequest of 15,000 pounds to the Hôtel-Dieu for the creation of three beds; the administrators decided to place them in the Salle Sainte-Anne, which an additional bequest of 4000 pounds enabled them to equip and decorate. Henceforth under the patronage of St Francis, this ward became the novitiate just before the Revolution, but remained unhealthy, badly ventilated and ill-lit: the level of the floor had already been raised twice in attempts to cure its dampness. By 1930 the health of the postulants was giving so much cause for concern that the novitiate was transferred to the upper floor of the large wing. The Salle Sainte-Anne is now smaller than it was in the Middle Ages, partitions having been used to create a utility room and a corridor linking the main courtyard with a small rear courtyard.

Situated one above the other, the St John the Baptist and Notre Dame wards disappeared in 1645 when the floor separating them was removed to allow for the creation of a new 12-bed ward: the Salle Saint-Hugues, which an initially anonymous donor – in fact Hugues Bétauld, from Beaune, mentioned above – had offered to equip and finance. The decision to "break the floor" was taken in the interests of providing sufficient air for the new ward. The Franciscan monks authorised the opening of five tall arched windows on the monastery side, which made it possible to close off the lay-lights giving onto the medieval infirmary. The artist Isaac Moillon decorated the wall and ceiling with paintings to the glory of Saint-Hugues (St Hugh), the donor's patron saint. When the issue of

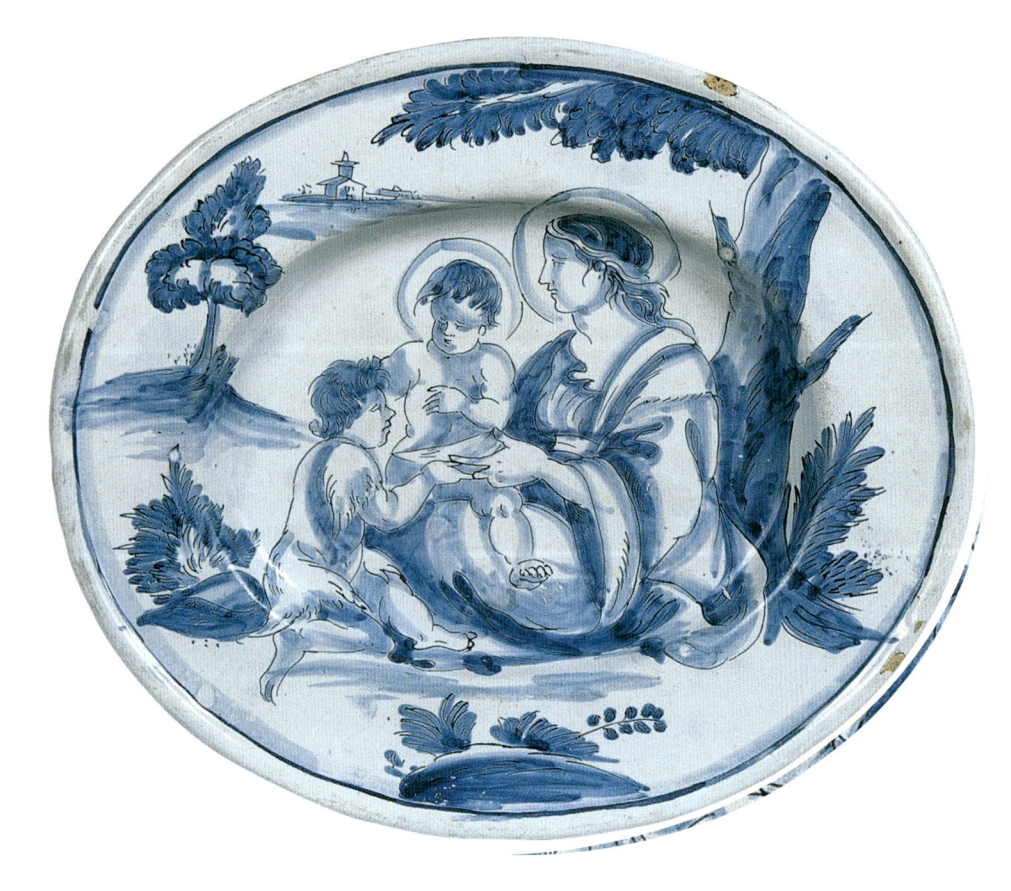

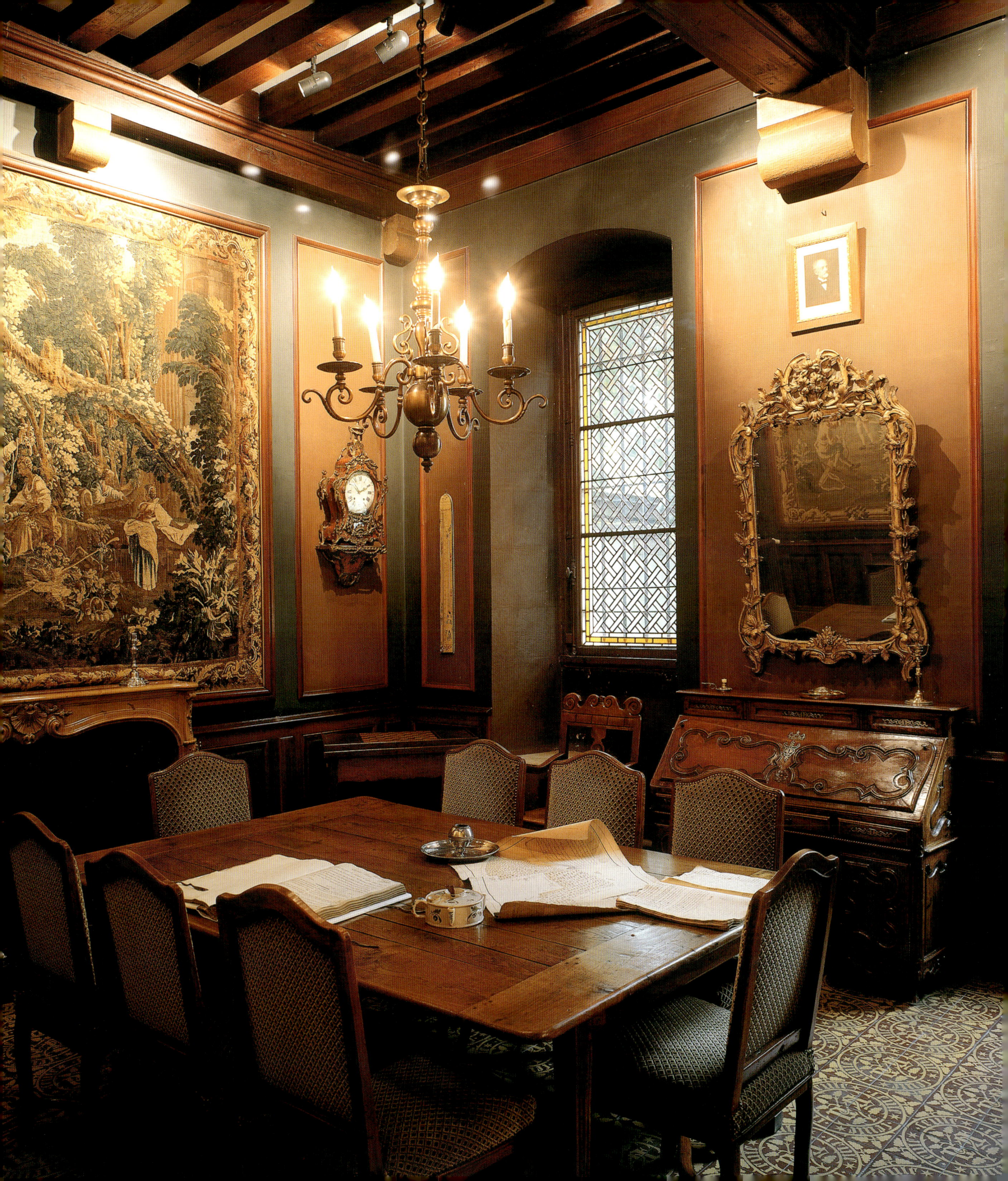

■ Below: The covered passage leading to the second courtyard.
Facing page: The Chambre-Dieu hagioscope seen from the chapel.

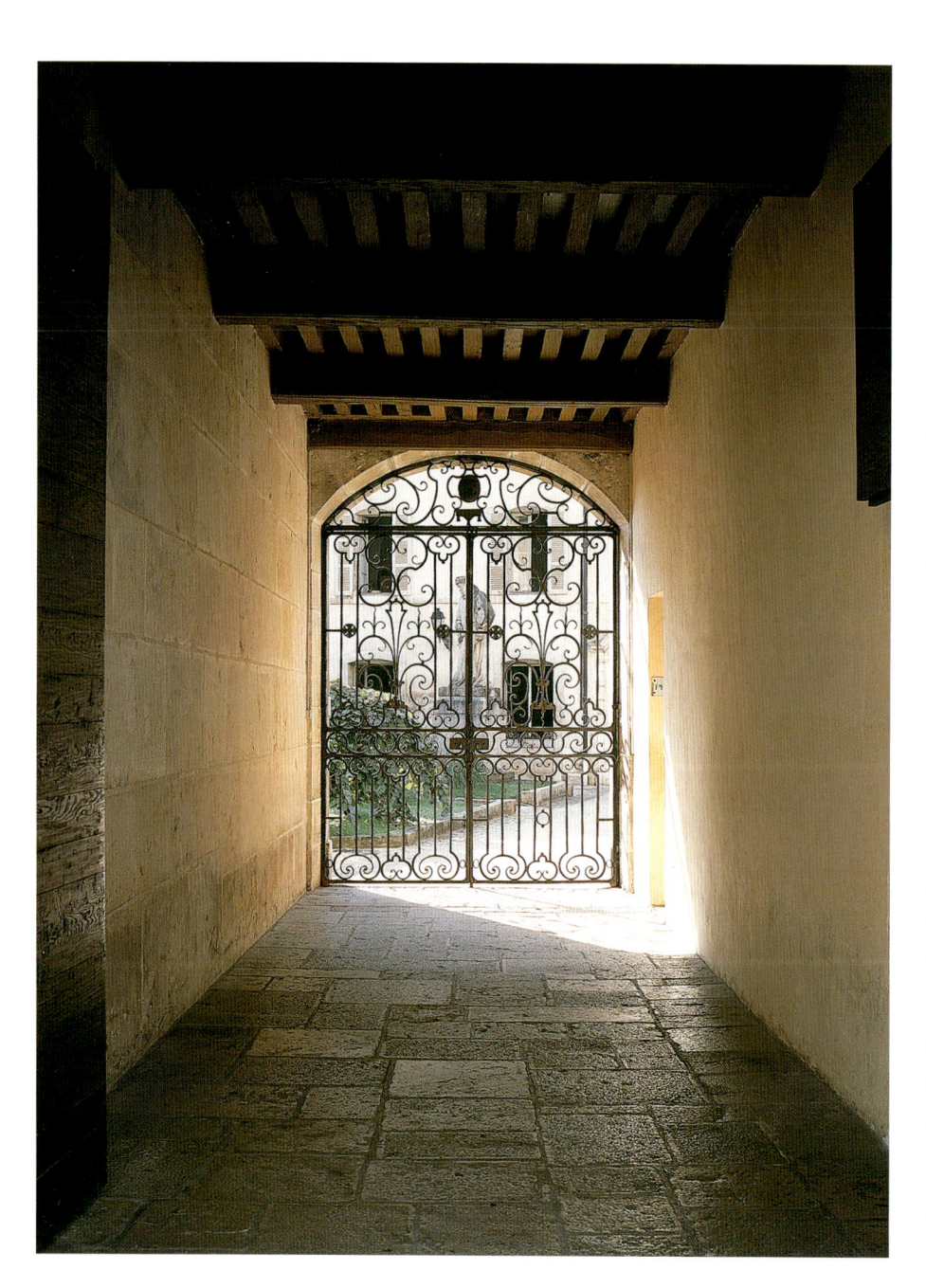

separating the sexes arose after the visit of Louis XIV, the men being cared for in the Great Hall were transferred in 1661 into this ward, where they enjoyed the comfort provided by an enormous open fire.

The Salle Sainte-Catherine, on the upper floor of the large courtyard wing, disappeared in 1784 at the same time as the Salle Sainte-Marthe on the ground floor. Their demolition, together with that of the two adjoining rooms – the medieval laundry and the nuns' workroom – made possible the creation of a new 12-bed ward financed, yet again, by an anonymous donor. Once again, for this new ward to be large and airy enough, the intervening floor had to be "broken". Also done away with was the passageway crossing the wing along the length of the kitchen and giving access, since the Middle Ages, to the gardens and cemetery. It was replaced with a new one, near the pharmacy: wider, more practical and closed off by a handsome wrought iron grille, it gave onto the granary. However, even though it had been provided with eight beds, the funds for fully equipping it were lacking and the new ward remained closed until the military strife of the Revolutionary period, when the Commissioner for War in Besançon required the Hôtel-Dieu, in 1793, to take in the sick and wounded of the army of the Rhine. The new Salle Notre-Dame, the third to bear the name, disappeared in turn in 1886-91, in the course of a vast reorganisation leading to the creation of a meeting room and offices followed, later on, by a small museum.

Situated at the end of the upper gallery, the Chambre-Dieu possessed a hagioscope, an aperture in the wall giving onto the chapel in the Great Hall and allowing the patient occupying the room to follow the daily offices. Renovated in 1785, when its windows were enlarged, and again at a later date, the Chambre-Dieu is now a storeroom, with no trace remaining of the "study" – the library – in its vestibule. In 1501, in addition to a number of breviaries and fine manuscript volumes, the library contained 65 books, all of them religious with the exception of several medical works – including three by the famous Persian doctor Avicenna (980-1037). Another 41 books were listed for the private rooms, among them a work on parchment "with drawings and accounts of herbs". The "study", to the east and next to the chapel, is reminiscent of the *armarium* found in Cistercian abbeys, usually set beside the church on the eastern aisle of the cloister. As late as 1880 it was still home to the hospitallers' library. Among the private rooms listed in 1501, two, situated one above the other, enjoyed undeniably special status: these were "the large ground-floor room over the river" and, above it, the Chambre de la Croix or Room of the Cross. Together they occupied the western end of the large courtyard wing, looking out onto the river Bouzaise. Sumptuously furnished, each possessed a smaller utility room and a toilet on its river side; on the ground floor these latter were set beneath ribbed vaults. In his accounts dating from the beginning of the building of the two rear wings,

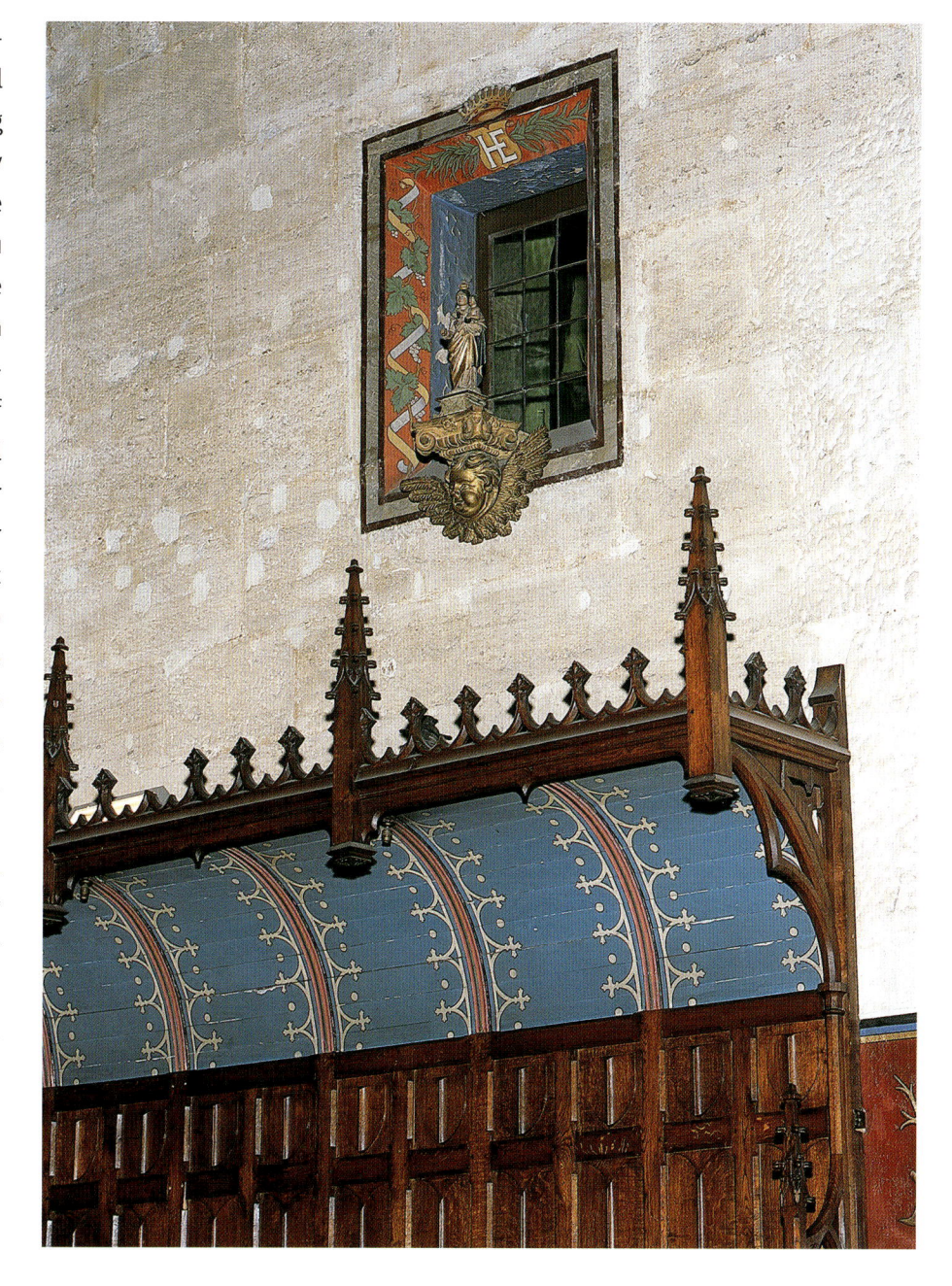

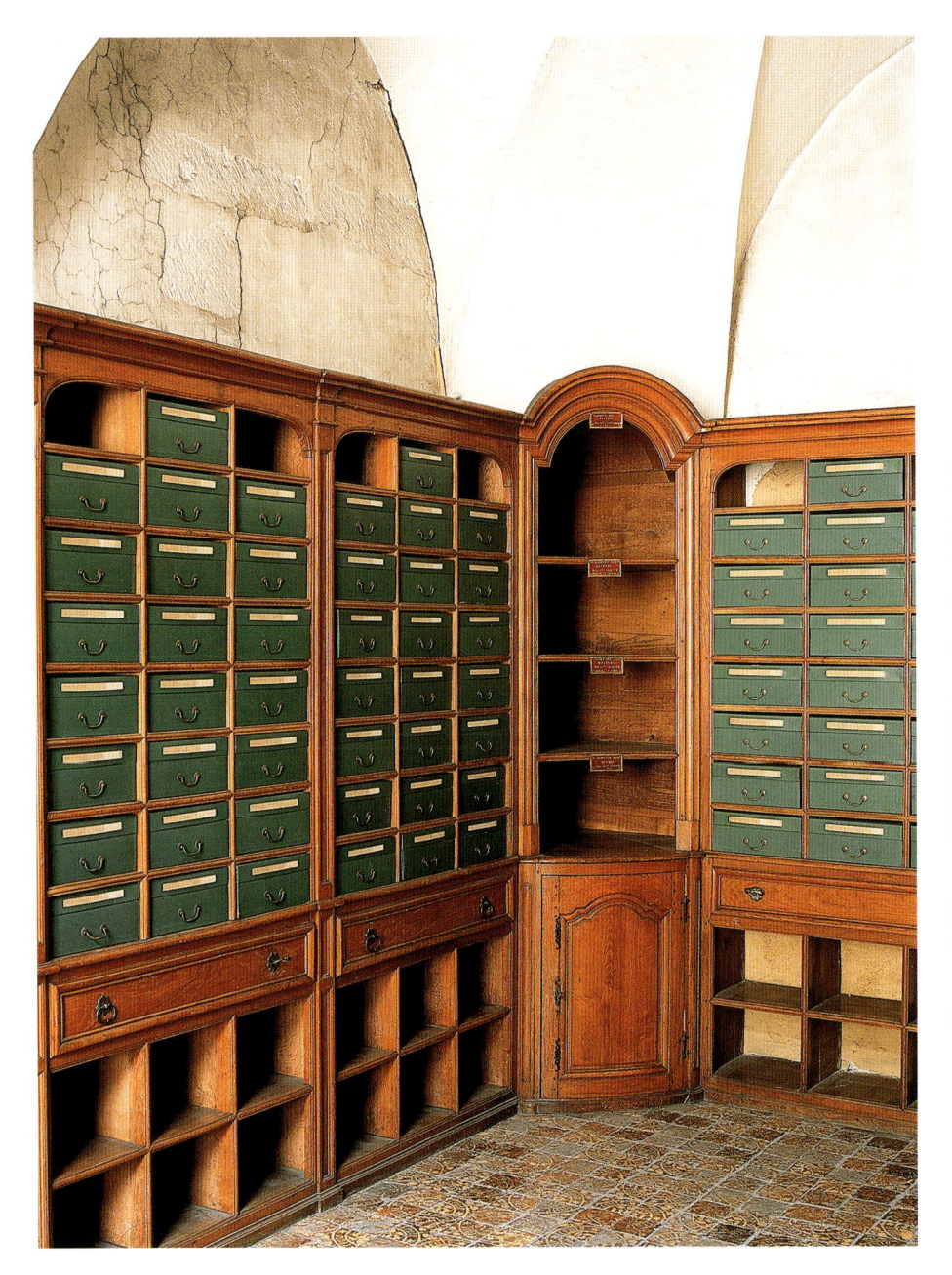

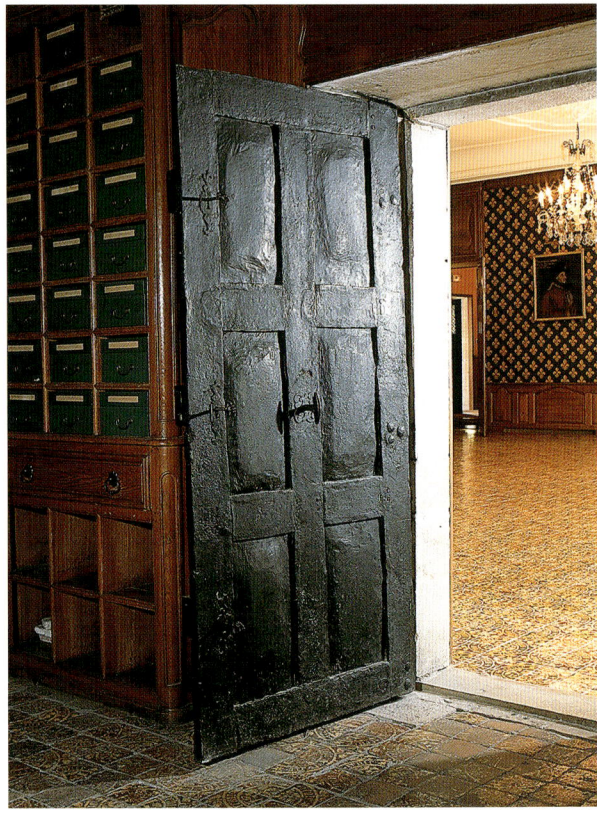

■ Above: The archives, designed in the 18th century.
Above right: The door of the archives.

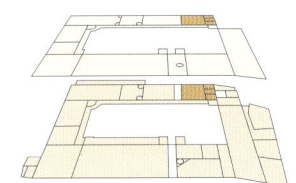

notary Jehannot Bar makes mention of the "Chambre Madame" – clearly "the large ground-floor room over the river" of the 1501 inventory and the quarters of Guigone de Salins. This room would later become the pharmacy.

All the indications are that the Room of the Cross was Nicolas Rolin's quarters, but the accounts covering the building of the upper floor are lacking. Agreeably situated and extremely well lit thanks to its large dormer window and windows opening south-wards onto a "little garden", it was certainly the most prestigious accommodation in the Hôtel-Dieu. After all, had it not been used by King Charles VIII at various times between 1484-98? In memory of these visits it was renamed the Chambre du Roi or the King's Room, and seems to have served mainly as an official drawing room until becoming a meeting room for the board of directors in 1745-48. Renovated in the style of the period, the original room was now unrecognisable, with its fireplace and Louis XV panelling, its medieval beams plastered over and its windows enlarged. Its two adjoining small rooms were knocked together to provide secure storage for the hospital's archives and money, their exposed-joist ceiling being covered, for fire safety reasons, with a groined vault of plastered brick. A solid door equipped with three locks and an external cladding of sheet iron discouraged unwanted visitors. By 1875 the archives had grown to the point where a carpenter was called in to install 108 shelves. Late in the 19th century the directors decided to transfer their meetings to the former Salle Notre-Dame on the ground floor, but the archives stayed put.

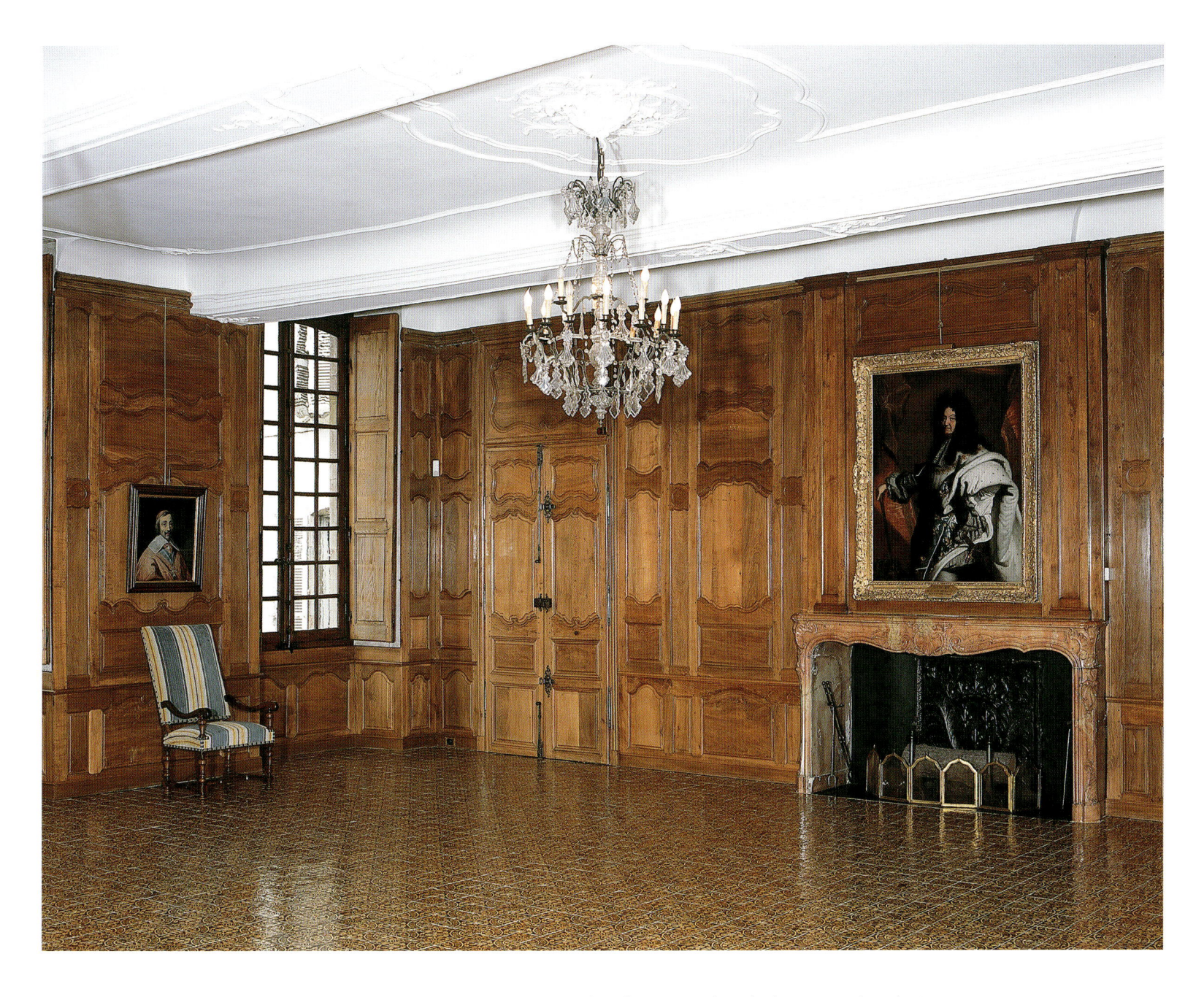

THE KITCHEN

While no study has yet been made of patient nutrition at the Hôtel-Dieu, research carried out in similar hospitals has revealed a concern with providing a

▌ Above: The King's Room, which in the 18th century became a meeting room for the board of directors.
Following page:
The kitchen.

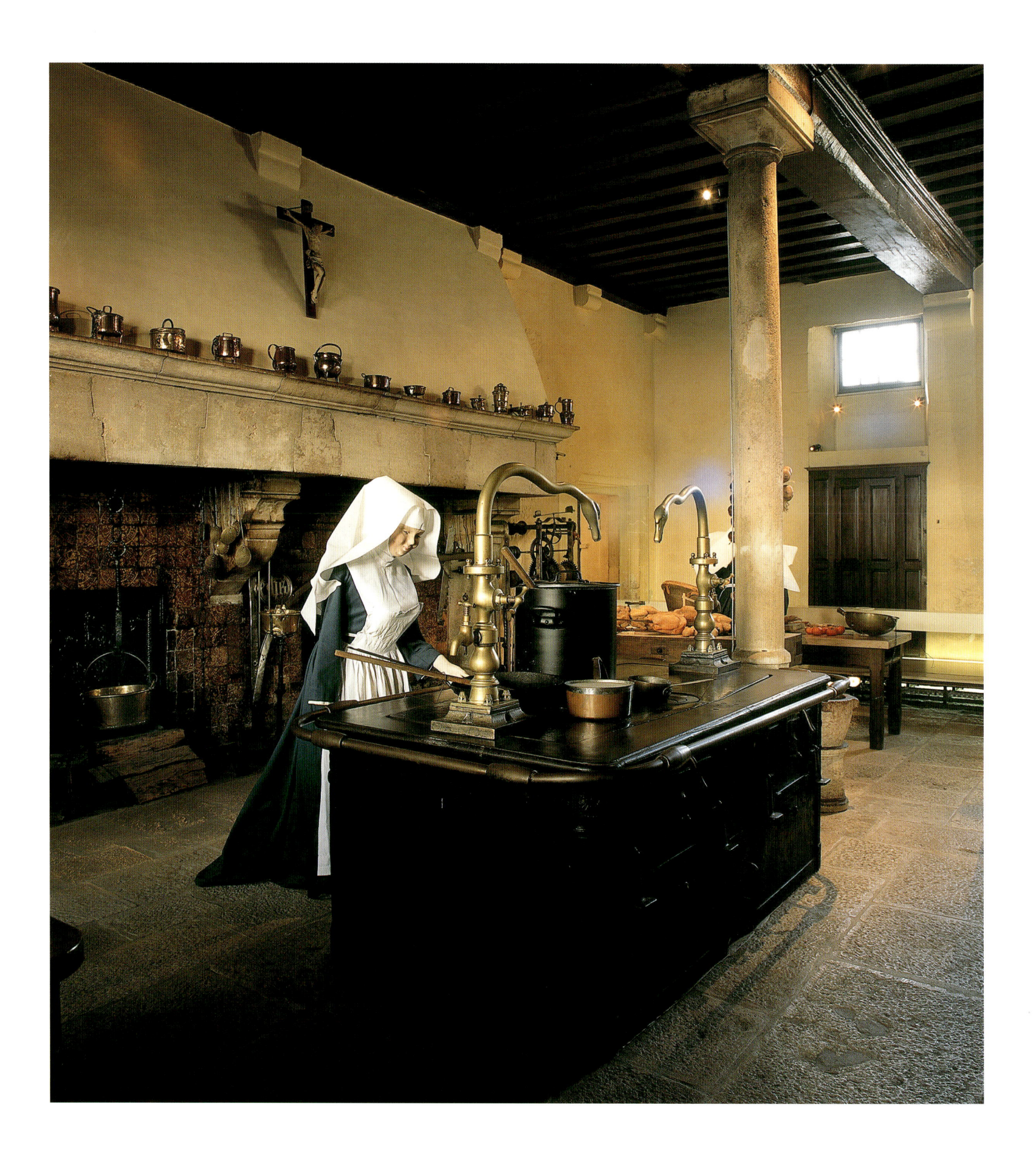

relatively balanced diet, giving patients food they liked and ensuring a supply of certain vegetables. Conversely, there was a regrettable tendency to overfeed the dying. When the Hôtel-Dieu opened, its enormous kitchen had to prepare meals for 86 sick poor, plus the sick from the private rooms, the nuns, their confessor, the two chaplains, and three servants from the hospital farm: all in all, some 130 people. The kitchen had a wide, double-hearth, in-wall fireplace, each hearth having its own function: as is still the case, the slightly larger one on the right was occupied by a triple spit, overhauled in 1697-98 by a clockmaker named Dufresne, who embellished it with the little wooden figure known as My Lord Bertrand. The other hearth was home to "two cauldrons for heating water", each with a copper lid "to keep the water hot longer". In 1756 the fireback and flue were partly demolished, rebuilt and connected to the chimney in the second infirmary. They were remodelled in 1781 after three chimney fires in quick succession.

In the middle of the kitchen two slender stone columns supported the exposed-joist ceiling. The records inform us that one of these columns, "very close to the fireplace", was put in place in 1469, apparently to replace a prop installed ten years earlier, when the beam had broken and the floor above collapsed.

The turrets overhanging two corners of the kitchen have neither the same function nor the same age. The one on the gallery side conceals a staircase, not part of the original building, leading to the nuns' infirmary. The first mention of the other – as a storage place for wood – is on a plan dating from 1903.

In 1754 a row of small utility rooms with groined vault ceilings was built against the facade giving onto the garden. They partially blocked the windows and made the kitchen so dark that in 1802 it was decided to enlarge the windows on the courtyard side. The kitchen sink is a replica of the original.

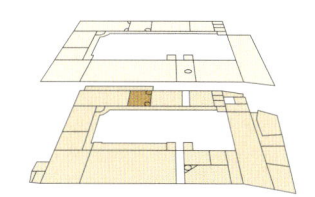

THE OVENS AND THE FLOUR STORE

The two ovens in the "oven room" next-door to the kitchen were kept permanently alight, being used not only for bread-making, but also for cooking the Hôtel-Dieu's "commons". A communicating door to the right of the fireplace meant there was no need to use the gallery. Before and after baking sessions, loaves and dishes were lined up on three big tables. This was also where the dough was kneaded, the flour being stored in the room directly above. These ovens disappeared in 1754 when the women's infirmary was created; in turn the new ovens, installed in a house next to the Hôtel-Dieu and facing the covered market, were transferred in 1827 to the ground floor of the granary, to allow for extension of the Salle Saint-Louis.

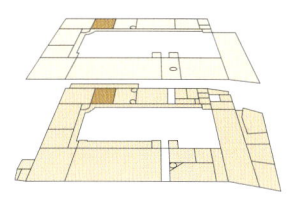

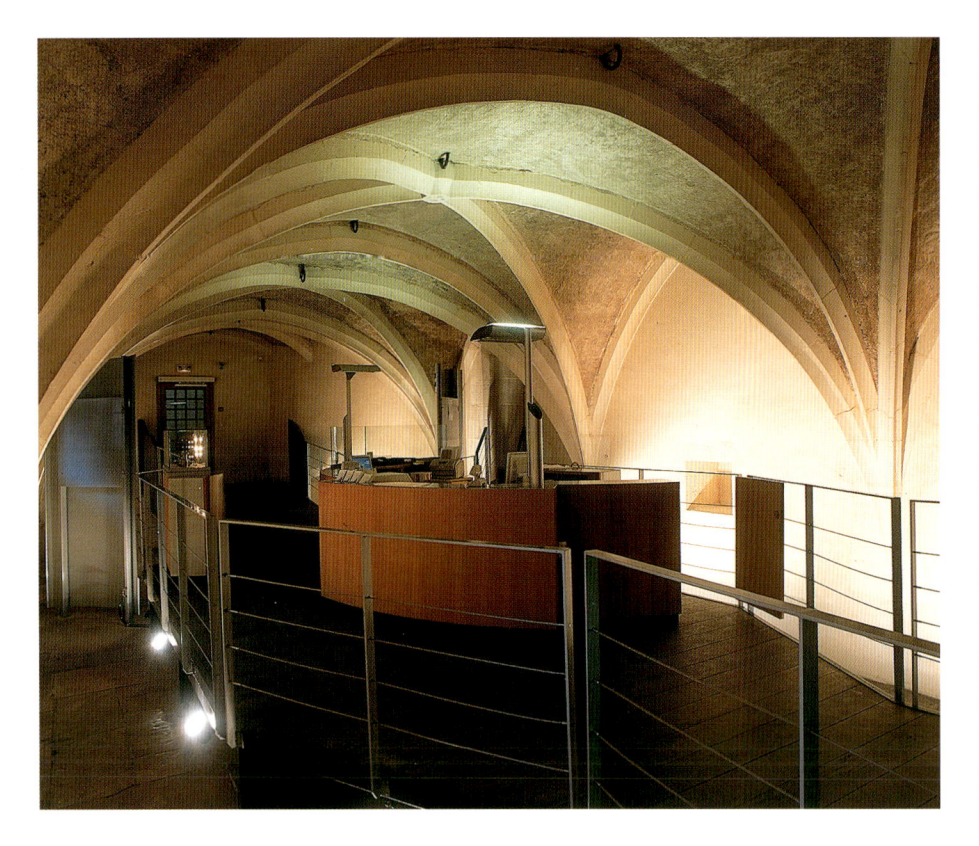

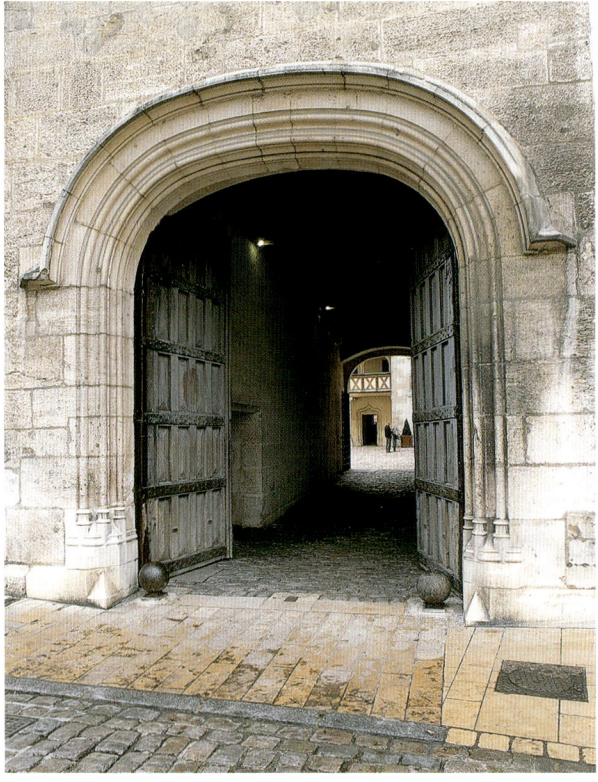

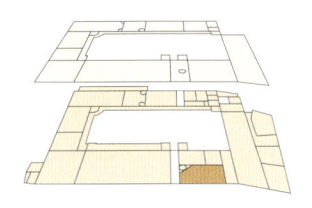

Above: The former refectory cellar, now the ticket office.
Above right: The coach and cart entrance.

THE REFECTORY CELLAR

The inventory of 1501 paints a picture of food stored here, there and everywhere. For the staff this meant endless comings and goings across the courtyard, especially between the kitchen and the main wing on the street, either to get to the "refectory cellar" or to climb the spiral staircase to the granary, where the nuns stored wheat, peas, fava beans, chickpeas, rice, barley and ground oats. Then there were the daily trips to the cheese store over the kitchen: in 1501 the store contained six dozen cheeses and a thousand eggs, the latter doubtless laid by the 40 or so hens at the hospital farm on Rue Paradis. Close to 1500 litres of vinegar were stored in the garden gallery. Next-door to the ovens, a little room called a *chambrote* housed the precious salt brought from Salins, in the Jura, at the express desire of the donor. It was transported using a large canvas tarpaulin and eight sacks of different sizes. The only survivor of all these storerooms, apart from the granary, is the "refectory cellar", set on the street as far as possible from the river. It is now the ticket office. In 1501 this cellar with its four ribbed vaults housed 25 barrels of wine – some 11,250 litres in all – and two stone troughs containing 300 litres of oil. There was also a little olive oil, together with bacon, candles, blocks of tallow and leather "for soling the sisters' shoes". The well that was still there in 1887 was so polluted, notably by the local tripe and offal butchers, that it had become "unthinkable to use its water for washing the dishes". Streetside the cellar was lit by four little square windows with wrought iron grilles, one of which bore a curious little "collection box for the patients of the Hôtel-Dieu", into which passers-by could drop a coin. Directly under the eye of the nuns, the cellar communicated with their refectory; however the barrels and deliveries were brought in via a door that the carters arriving on the square in front of the covered market found immediately on their left, under the covered passageway. The very medieval-looking door separating the visitors' entry hall from the former cellar – now the ticket office – dates in fact from 1873, when access was needed to the porter's lodge then being built in the corner of the cellar.

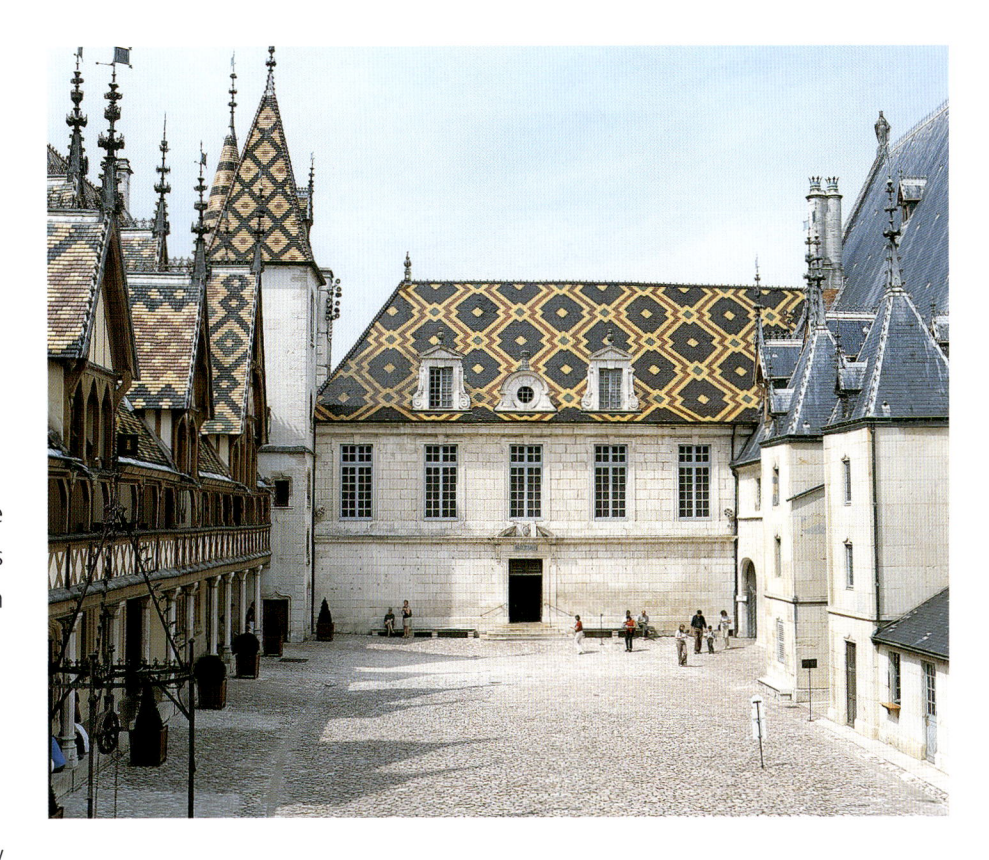

THE WINEPRESS HOUSE

Situated to the west of the courtyard on the site now occupied by the Salle Saint-Louis, the building housing the winepress was completed in 1469, seven years after Nicolas Rolin's death. The 1501 inventory makes mention of a "handsome" lever-operated press, together with seven large and five smaller vats providing a total capacity of 16,700 litres. The list of equipment points to a fairly large building, and in fact a second press was installed at a later date. An upper floor served as storage space for bundles of vine shoots, metal hoops for barrels, and willow for weaving grape-harvest baskets. A "cellar" contained winemaking equipment, but no barrels.

In 1660 the directors voted to replace the press house with a twelve-bed ward which Louis Bétauld, brother of the founder of the Salle Saint-Hugues, undertook to finance. As an economy measure, it was decided not to demolish the press house completely, but rather to retain all or part of the walls not visible from the courtyard. The roof structure was also reused, at least partially. Built over the river, the new-ward was likely to be damp, so the ground floor was raised. A utility building at the back gave access to the still uncovered part of river, into which the nuns emptied the patients' bedpans.

In accordance with its founder's wish, the cut stone courtyard facade resembles that of the Great Hall of the Poor. Like all the rooms intended for a large number of patients, this one was high and airy, and was lit by five large windows that were closed off in the 20th century. By today's standards the chimney might seem small for the space it had to heat, but the original Salle Saint-Louis was only half the present size: in 1827-29 it was extended as far as the street, after demolition of the ovens and the house of the chaplains, whose new quarters were in an adjoining building. Except for the tall, wide, arched windows giving onto the square, this extension matched the style of the initial ward. It now contained 26 beds exclusively for military patients, for whom a free-standing fountain of polished Ladoix stone was installed. The paintings ornamenting the fireplace, showing the coats of arms of Nicolas Rolin, Guigone

▌ Above: The Salle Saint-Louis, built in the 17th century on the former site of the barn housing the winepress.

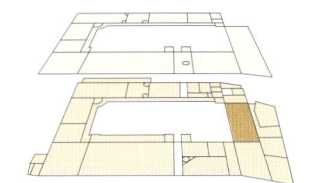

de Salins and Louis Bétauld, and the frieze that highlights the exposed-joist ceiling all date from the early 20th century. In 1974 the famous *Last Judgement* polyptych, commissioned from Rogier Van der Weyden by Nicolas Rolin, was installed in air-conditioned premises in the rear of the Salle Saint-Louis.

THE LAUNDRY AND OUTDOOR WASH-HOUSE

In spite of the obvious inconvenience it caused, the laundry where the nuns boiled up the linen was between two rooms, one of them that of Guigone de Salins. After visiting in 1619, a certain Father Fodéré declared it "a fine big laundry, with the coppers cemented into a low wall of cut stone. The vats the linen is put into for steaming are round, handsome and also of cut stone, and laid out in such a way that the linen makes its own way there, via channels of the same kind of stone." After rinsing and wringing the linen on the stones of the wash-house, the nuns put it into baskets and carried their heavy load up one or other of the spiral staircases to the attics, where they hung it on wooden poles. This system was in use for a long time, as the many surviving poles attest. The laundry was pulled down in 1784. Demolition of the wash-house in 1854 meant the river could be covered and the site paved.

FROM DISPENSARY TO PHARMACY

For its founder the Hôtel-Dieu existed to cure illness; it was not at all a place where people went to die, the patients being cared for "until they had regained their health or reached convalescence." The archives testify to the presence of doctors in the 15th century, as well as surgeons and the barbers who filled in as surgeons. The records for the early 16th century mention a Beaune apothecary named Nicolas Richart, but there is no evidence that the dispensary inventoried in 1501 was there when the Hôtel-

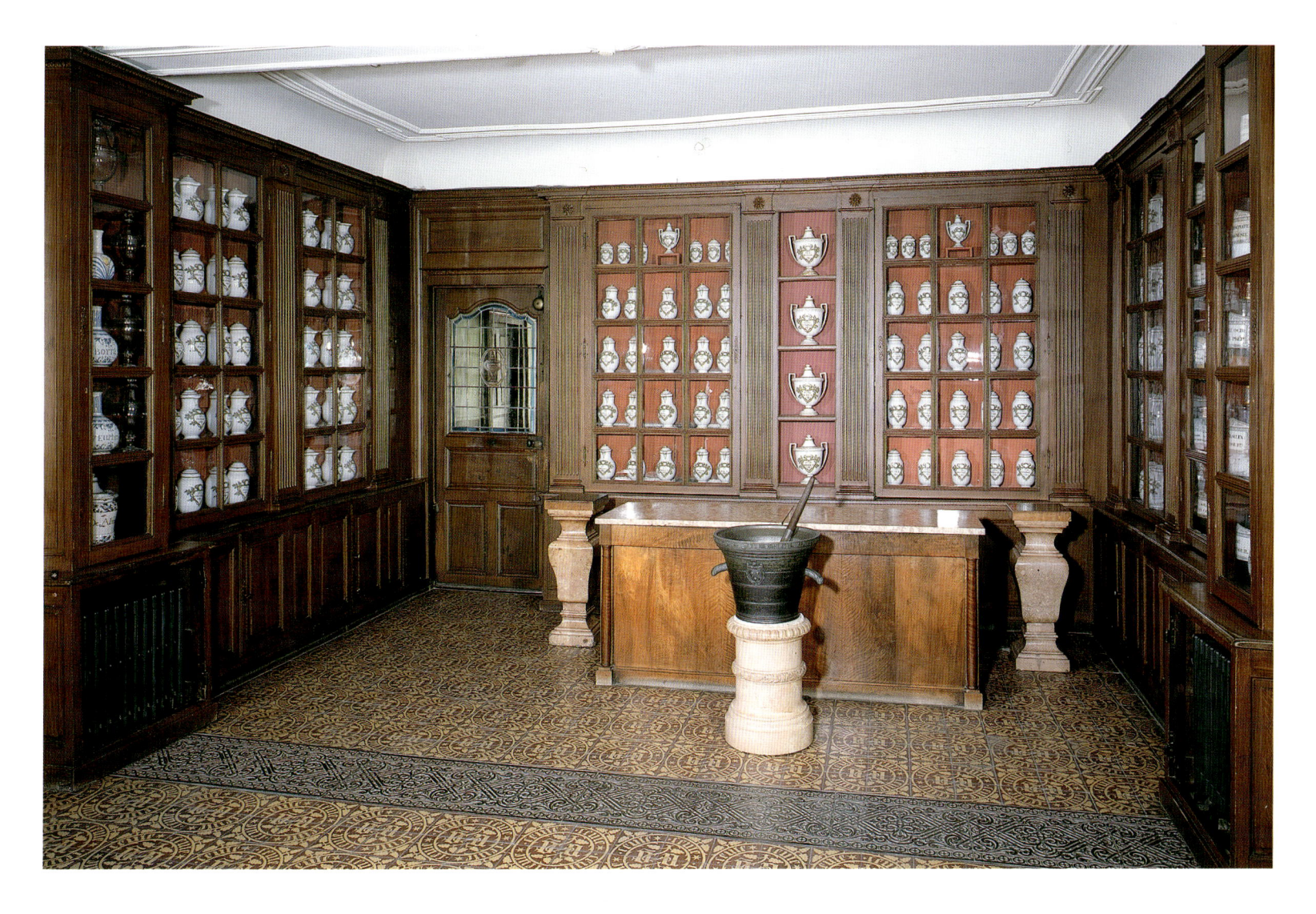

Dieu opened its doors on 1 January 1452. Its installation – curious to say the least – in one of the little utility rooms off Guigone de Salins' quarters, would seem to indicate the contrary. It may in fact date from the last decade of the 15th century, when France's big hospitals were beginning to employ their own apothecaries.

It would seem that a hundred or so phials of medicine were lined up on shelves, together with a dozen pewter containers for cordials and preserves, six glazed earthenware apothecary's pots for syrups and four lead boxes containing the famous universal antidotes theriac and mithridate. There were also two small vats, one filled with honey and the other with soap, and several *bruches* of different jams. The 17th century saw the arrival of special cupboards, whose little doors, decorated with painted flowers, can still be seen today. Until 1745 the dispensary and the room next-door, on the garden side, served as the "treasury", where money, precious items and the Hôtel-Dieu archives were kept.

With the pharmacopoeia constantly expanding, more and more space was needed, and in 1776 the directors decided to renovate the dispensary, which they found "enormous, ill-lit, cold and very uncomfortable". Clearly they were referring not to the medieval room, with its area of no more than 12 square metres, but to the former "ground floor room over the river", which had little by little been taken over by pharmaceutical supplies. Major changes – it

▌Facing page: Doors with flower decoration in the former dispensary. Above: The pharmacy, created in the 17th century.

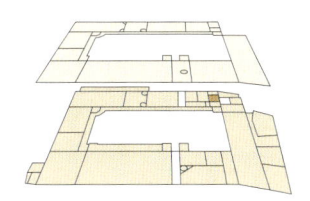

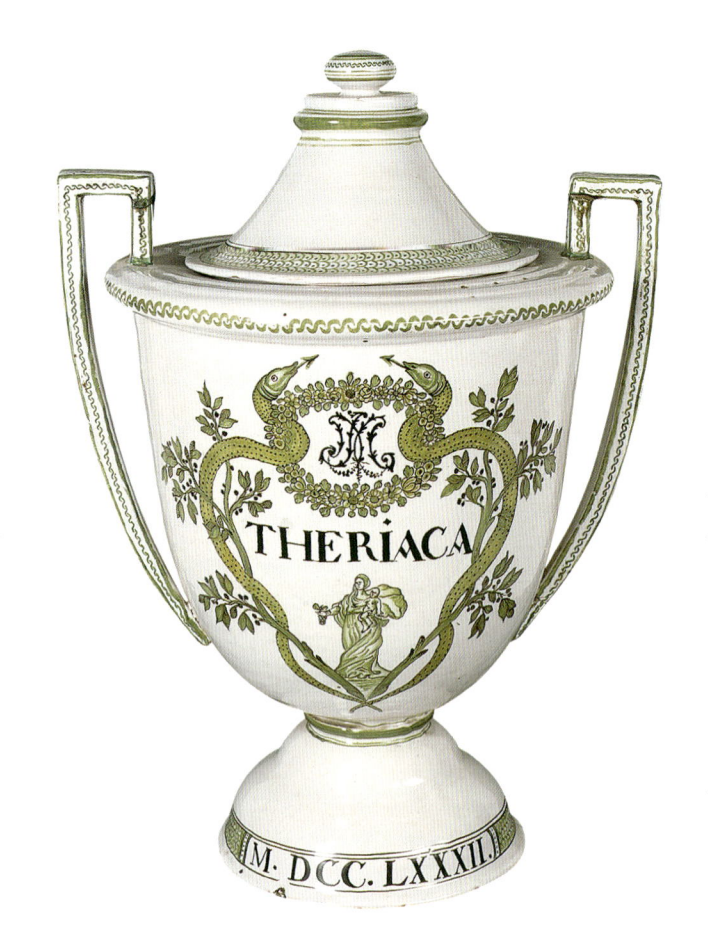

■ Right: Earthenware theriac pot dated 1782, probably from Franche-Comté.
Below: The laboratory, fitted out in the 19th century.

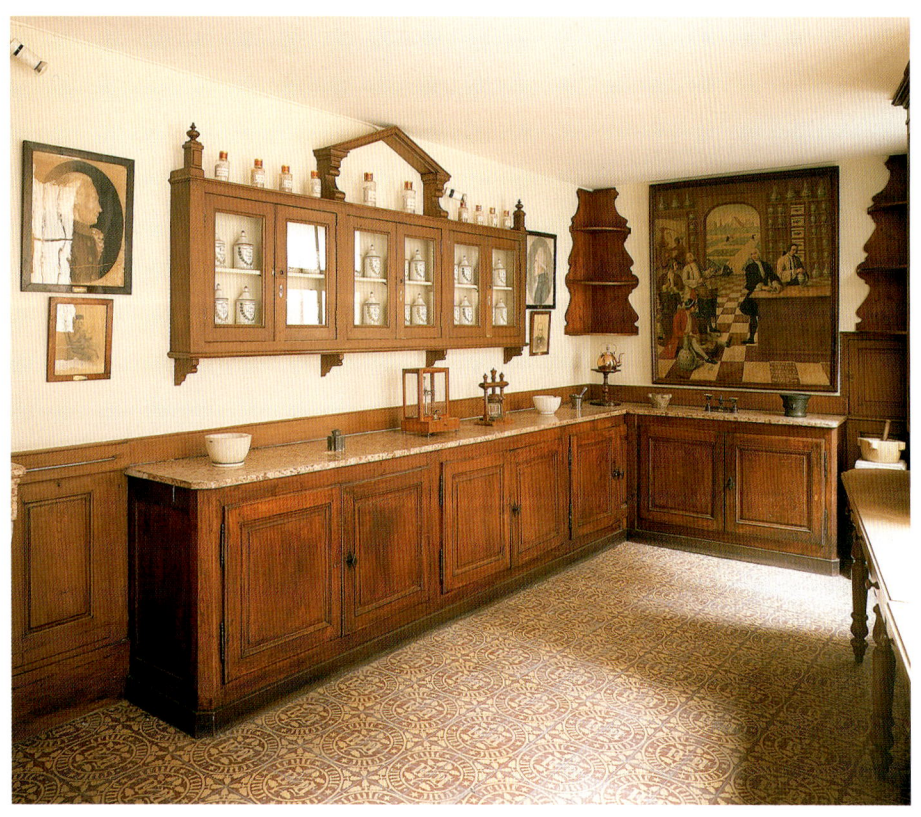

was partitioned into four rooms with a small vestibule that could be reached from the gallery – meant "the aforesaid room was rearranged in a way better suited to its role as dispensary". The medieval column holding up the central ceiling beam remained visible.

On the garden side a new pharmacy was set up, with a room for the hospitallers who worked there; and on the courtyard side two small rooms served as annexes. The creation of a fourth window, giving onto the garden, and enlargement of the three others brought in more air and light, while in the interests of unity and brightness the exposed-joist ceiling was plastered over. In 1787, doubtless to accommodate an order of pots, master carpenter Joseph Bonhomme was charged with providing "panelling and shelving for the dispensary". The resultant cupboards with their fluted pilasters are still in place today. Their installation, however, blocked off the medieval door leading to the former dispensary, which was replaced with a door giving access to what had once been the "treasury" and was now a laboratory. In 1819 a Ladoix stone fireplace replaced the original one, which dated from the building of the Hôtel-Dieu.

Paying an apothecary and purchasing ever-increasing quantities of medicine was an expensive business. The cost was supposed to be met by selling off clothing inherited from the patients, but the income was inadequate: as Sister Grozelier complained in

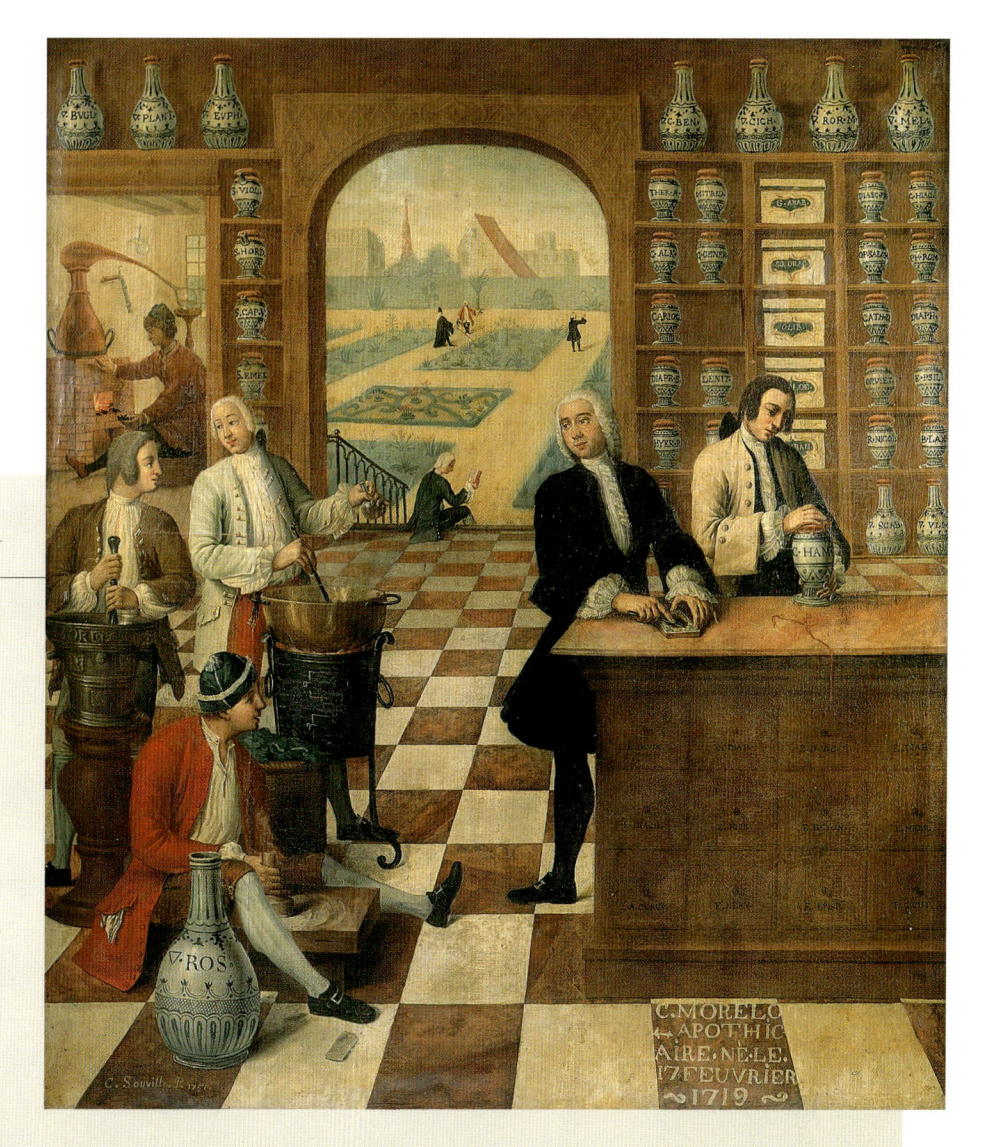

A mid-18th-century dispensary

In a painting from 1751 Charles Coquelet Souville portrays Claude Morelot at work at the Hôtel-Dieu dispensary. Elegantly clad in a black suit with lace ruffle and cuffs, the apothecary is kneading a pharmaceutical product with a spatula as his assistants busy themselves grinding, heating and distilling various medicines. Under the pretext of a genre portrait, the artist neatly captures the atmosphere of the dispensary, carefully detailing the spotless tiled floor, the blue-and-white pots on the shelves and the meticulously labelled drawers. Off the dispensary is the laboratory, where a copper alembic is being heated, while a central doorway giving onto the simples garden reminds us of the vital role of medicinal plants in the pharmacopoeia of the period.

The overall composition is borrowed from an etching by the Dutch engraver Jacobus Harrewijn which had served as the frontispiece for the 1702 *Pharmacopée de Bruxelles*, a work Morelot doubtless had a copy of. However, Souville adapted the original to its new context by including, in addition to Morelot's portrait, a mortar bearing his name – and which resembles the tinned bronze mortar on a pink marble base Morelot had had made in 1760 and which can still be seen in the Hôtel-Dieu pharmacy. The mortar bears its owner's coat of arms, an inscription mentioning his rank of assistant medical officer in the army and the name of his wife, Claudine Léger. The accompanying pestle is so heavy it had to be operated mechanically, using an arch-shaped device attached to the ceiling.

▊ *Claude Morelot in his dispensary*, C. Souville, 1751.

■ Above and facing page: The nuns' refectory, refurbished in the 18th century.

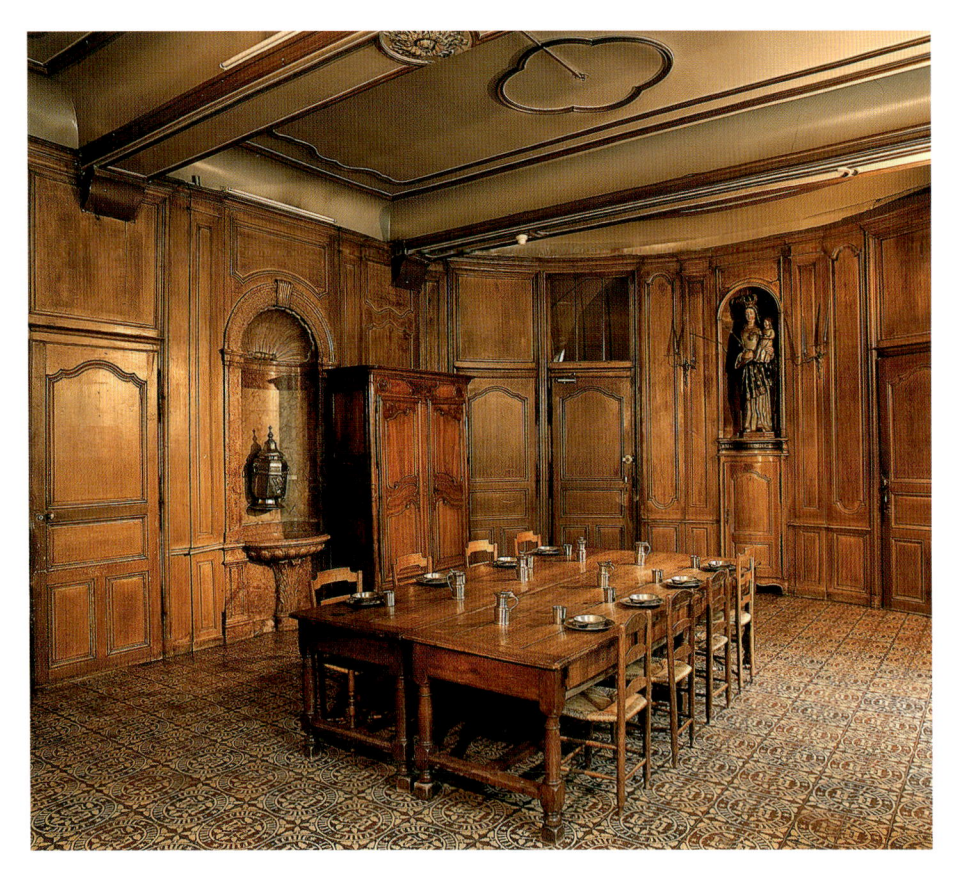

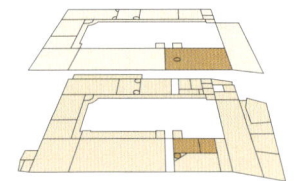

1774, "The revenue from what is left by deceased patients is decreasing steadily because of their practice of arriving with very small quantities of wretched clothing." It was decided in 1788 to dispense with the apothecary's services and train two resident staff as pharmacists. On the point of closing his dispensary, the apothecary Gremeau undertook their training and sold the Hôtel-Dieu his equipment, which included the large collection of earthenware pots, decorated with snakes and green glaze, that are still a feature of the pharmacy window. The archives do not give the pots' place of origin, but they would seem to be from the Franche-Comté region in eastern France. Once trained, the nun-pharmacists began selling their medicines, but as business increased their premises became cramped. In 1820 the donation of a stable and a small yard on the tripe butchers' alley made room for a long, narrow but larger laboratory with three tall windows.

THE NUNS' ROOMS

The community of hospitaller nuns had four rooms set aside for it: a refectory and dormitory under the same roof as the Great Hall, and across the courtyard, on the upper floor of the large wing, an infirmary and a workroom.

At midday and seven in the evening the nuns went to the refectory via the entry vestibule. There they took their meals on a long table whose wooden top, covered with a linen cloth, rested on "eight stone pillars". Six religious paintings softened the austere aspect of the cut stone walls. An adjoining room, the "little refectory", was used as an annexe. To wash the pewter, wood and terra cotta kitchenware the nuns had to go into the courtyard: "The sisters, lay sisters and postulants had always scoured the dishes on a little wooden bench by the small well outside the refectory; the well had never been provided with a roof to make this arduous task easier, and these young women were to be seen painfully at work come rain, frost or snow and in the hottest and coldest weather. Often their hands were swollen, but they were ready to work till they dropped without the slightest complaint."

Despite the poverty and asceticism imposed by their rule, the nuns were eventually provided with certain conveniences: in 1660 a wooden staircase was built inside the refectory, giving them direct access to the dormitory above. In 1776 the refectory was trans-

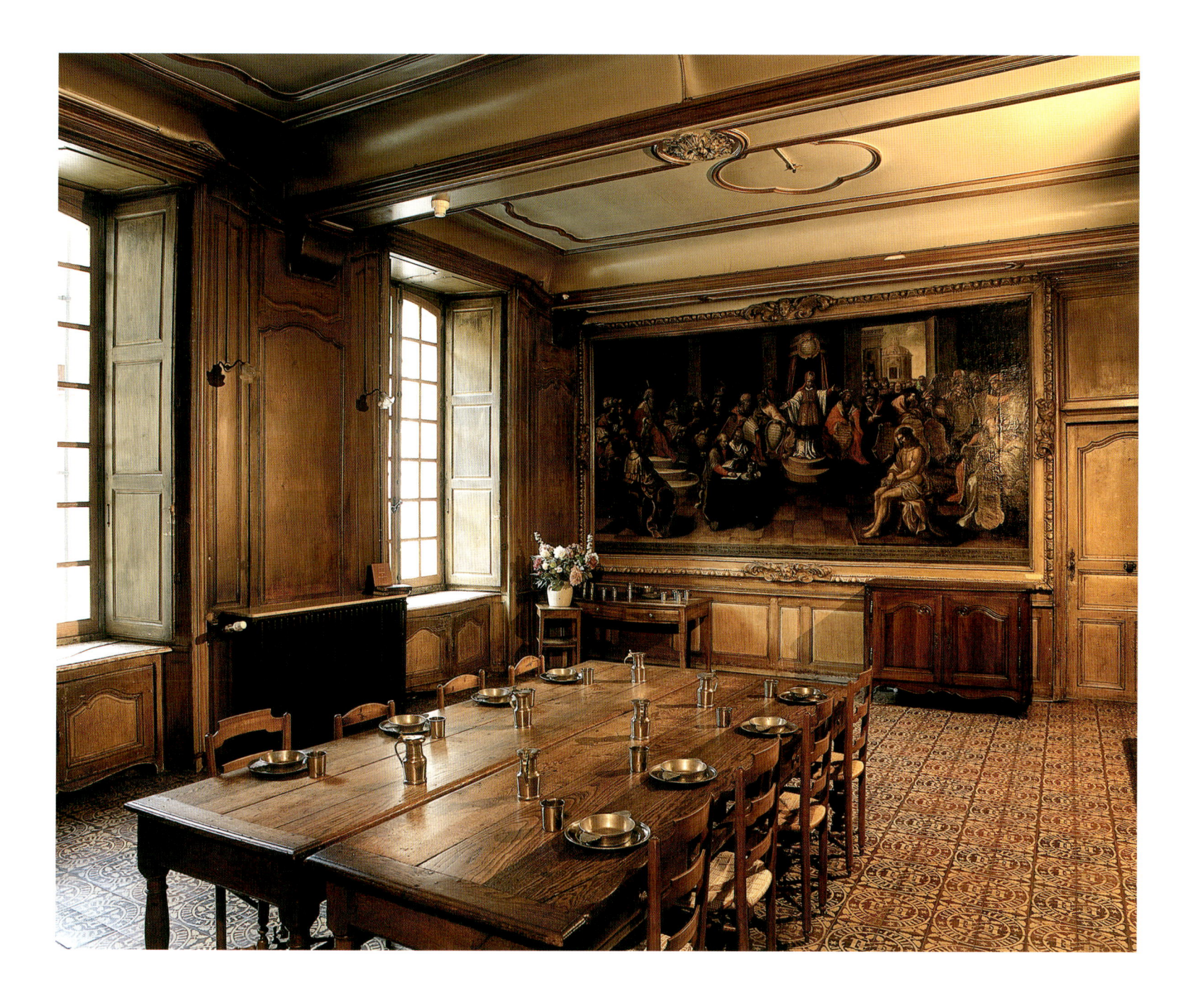

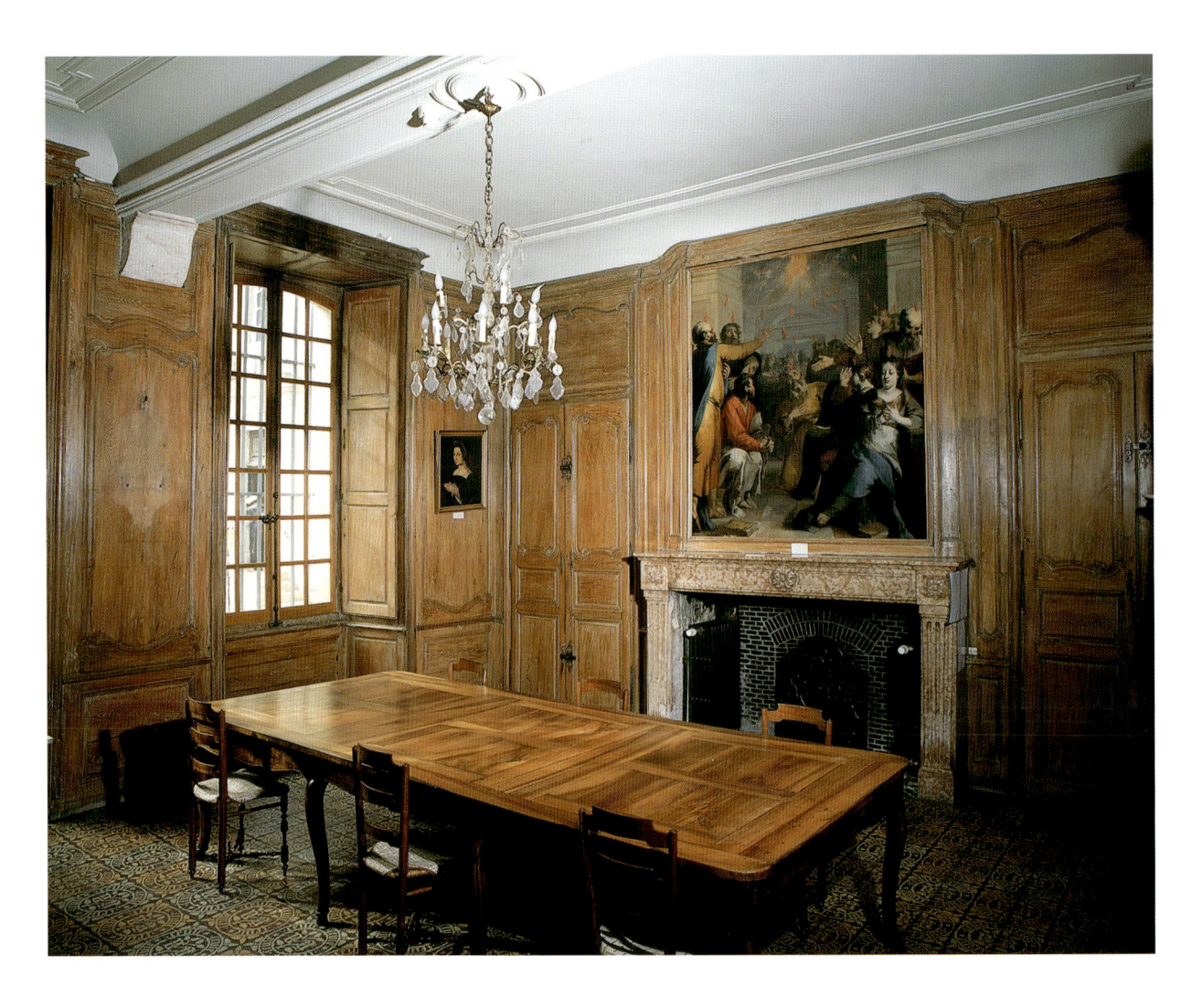

Right: The head nun's room, 18th century.
Facing page: Recreation of an alcove in the nuns' dormitory, 19th century.

formed at great expense, a new partition turning the little refectory into a larger room for the directress. The medieval windows were enlarged, tall wood panels hid the stone walls, and the dark beams disappeared under a plaster ceiling. A modern "Greek style" fireplace was installed in the directress's room and life was simplified by a fountain set in a half-domed niche decorated with a shell.

The little refectory was sorely missed, however, and in 1793 it was decided to create a small vaulted pantry by adding a pavilion in the courtyard, at the corner of the refectory. In the interest of "uniformity" another, symmetrically placed pavilion was built to serve as quarters for the doorman. Sixty years later the pavilions were raised to create two square turrets linked by a wooden walkway. As a result of this new arrangement the larder disappeared, making way for a staircase leading to the nuns' dormitory.

Sometime between eight and nine in the evening, the nuns climbed the spiral staircase which, in addition to leading to the dormitory, gave access to the attic and the belltower. At the time of the Hôtel-Dieu's founding a single dormitory probably sufficed, with its seventeen wooden beds behind their heavy curtains. Over the years, however, the community grew: by 1501 an extra six-bed dormitory and a small three-bed room had been added. The two dormitories had no heating – not even hot water bottles – but the 1501 inventory mentions a fireplace in the small bedroom, which was perhaps where the postulants slept.

Every night two nuns "took turns to watch over the sick in the infirmary and the hospital proper", but from the dormitory their companions were able to keep an eye on the Great Hall via two small windows, one in the middle of the partition wall and the other in the corner on the courtyard side. The centuries continued to pass and, apart from the 1660 staircase already mentioned, little effort was made to improve the level of comfort in the dormitories. In 1773, at the insistence of the doctors, it was decided to enlarge the windows giving onto the courtyard in the interests of better ventilation, but this concern with hygiene did not extend to "disfiguring" the streetside facade, whose windows were spared all modification. It was in 1819-20, as part of a large-scale renovation involving demolition of the wooden partitions, that the twenty-two alcoves to be seen today were installed. The former dormitory is now a storeroom.

The nuns' infirmary and workroom had fireplaces: a privilege for those who were ill or engaged in needlework. The Hôtel-Dieu's designer had also seen to it that the infirmary was over the kitchen, where the fire never went out. Sick nuns were allowed to wear "open fronted robes with fur lining". In 1501 the infirmary contained seven beds arranged to provide their occupants with a view of the altar and its painting of the Resurrection; and a generous amount of furniture made this a much less spartan setting than the dormitory.

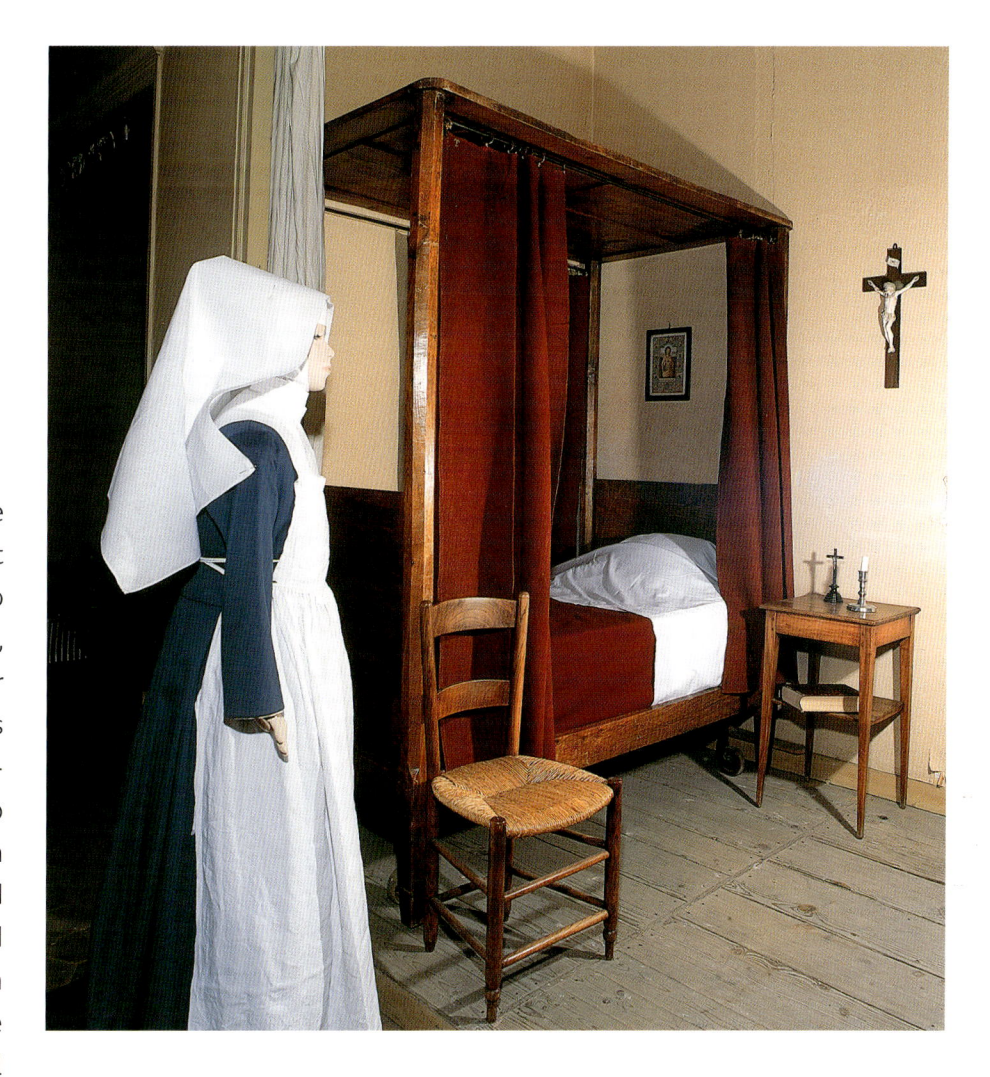

Off the infirmary, in the enormous workroom with its religious paintings, the nuns made clothes for the patients and for themselves, as well as the altar cloths and the bed and table linen. Cutting was done on a vast square table while sewing and embroidery – the inventory mentions a "locked wooden embroidery cabinet" – were done seated on a "long, low wooden dais" or on stools. Small looms were used for weaving fringes, ribbons and certain fabrics. All sorts of materials and linen were stored in the workroom, which also served as a wardrobe for storing clothes, the nuns' habits and the headdresses based on the tall, conical hennin worn by medieval noblewomen.

The infirmary and workroom have gone. In 1994-95 they were replaced, like the Salle Sainte-Catherine, with seminar rooms.

The garden extension and the cemetery

■ Below: The "granary", built in the 18th century. Facing page: The granary staircase.

South of the Hôtel-Dieu lay a large area of land occupied by the garden and a cemetery that included the "hospitallers' burial ground". A long gallery gave shelter from the weather and led to two small rooms for the "agitated patients" and a kind of mortuary chapel known as "the little room for burying the deceased". These buildings were still under way in 1469-71.

In the 17th century, at the time of Louis Bétauld's founding of the Salle Saint-Louis, shortage of space led the directors to construct new buildings in the garden. This was the beginning of ongoing extensions necessitating the acquisition of adjacent properties, initially for the creation of utility rooms and outbuildings. A granary had to be built in 1658-59, immediately followed by "a brand new building for the winepress and vats"; these replaced the medieval vat room supplanted in 1660 by the Salle Saint-Louis.

On the verge of collapse, the granary – an enormous three-storey building closing off the south side of the second courtyard – had to be rebuilt in 1736-38. The weight of the grain it housed meant vaulting the cellar, ground floor and first floor. Access to the upper floors was by a handsome, iron-railed staircase. The elegant panelled rendering of its façades was restored in 1989-90 on the winepress courtyard side.

Building the granary cut back the area of the cemetery, which soon turned out to be too small. At the time, with two or three hundred deaths every year, there was no choice but to "bury the dead very close together and open the graves again before the previous bodies were fully consumed". A proposal to buy land formerly occupied by the city's moats initially met with a flat refusal, the governor having planted willows there: it took a raid on the outskirts of Beaune by the famous bandit Mandrin, on 18 December 1754, to break the deadlock. The royal artillery was called in and the captain in charge judged it necessary to cut the willows down as they meant the moats could not be kept under surveillance. Thus the Hôtel-Dieu's new cemetery was blessed and opened on 27 August 1756.

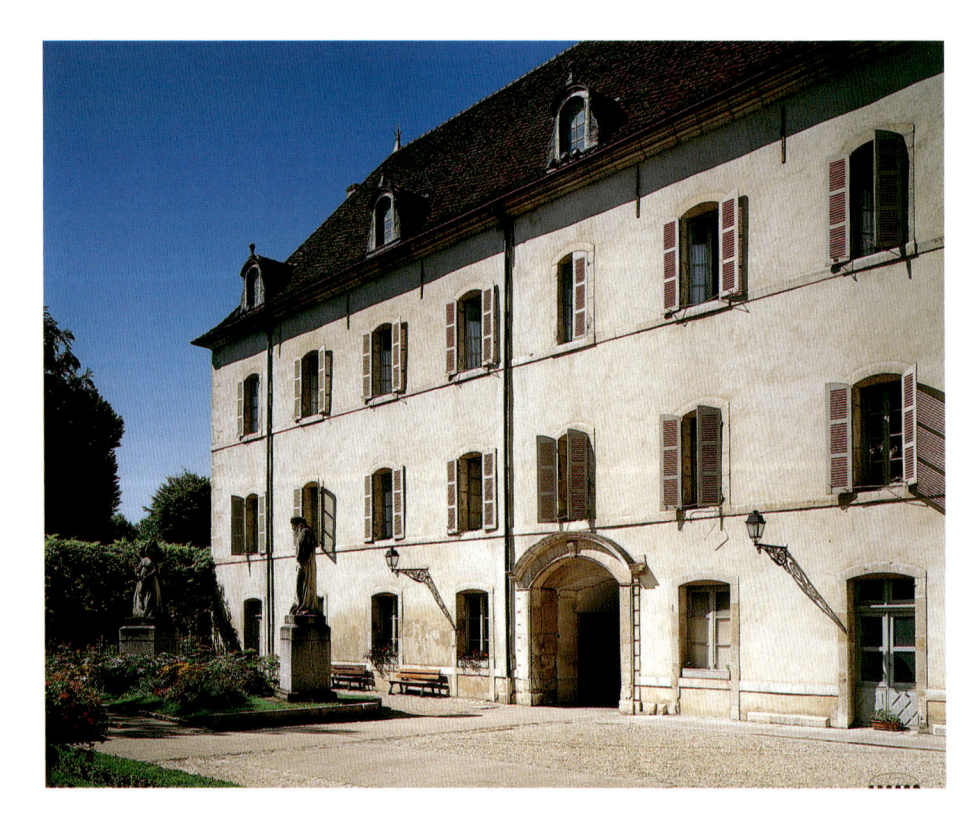

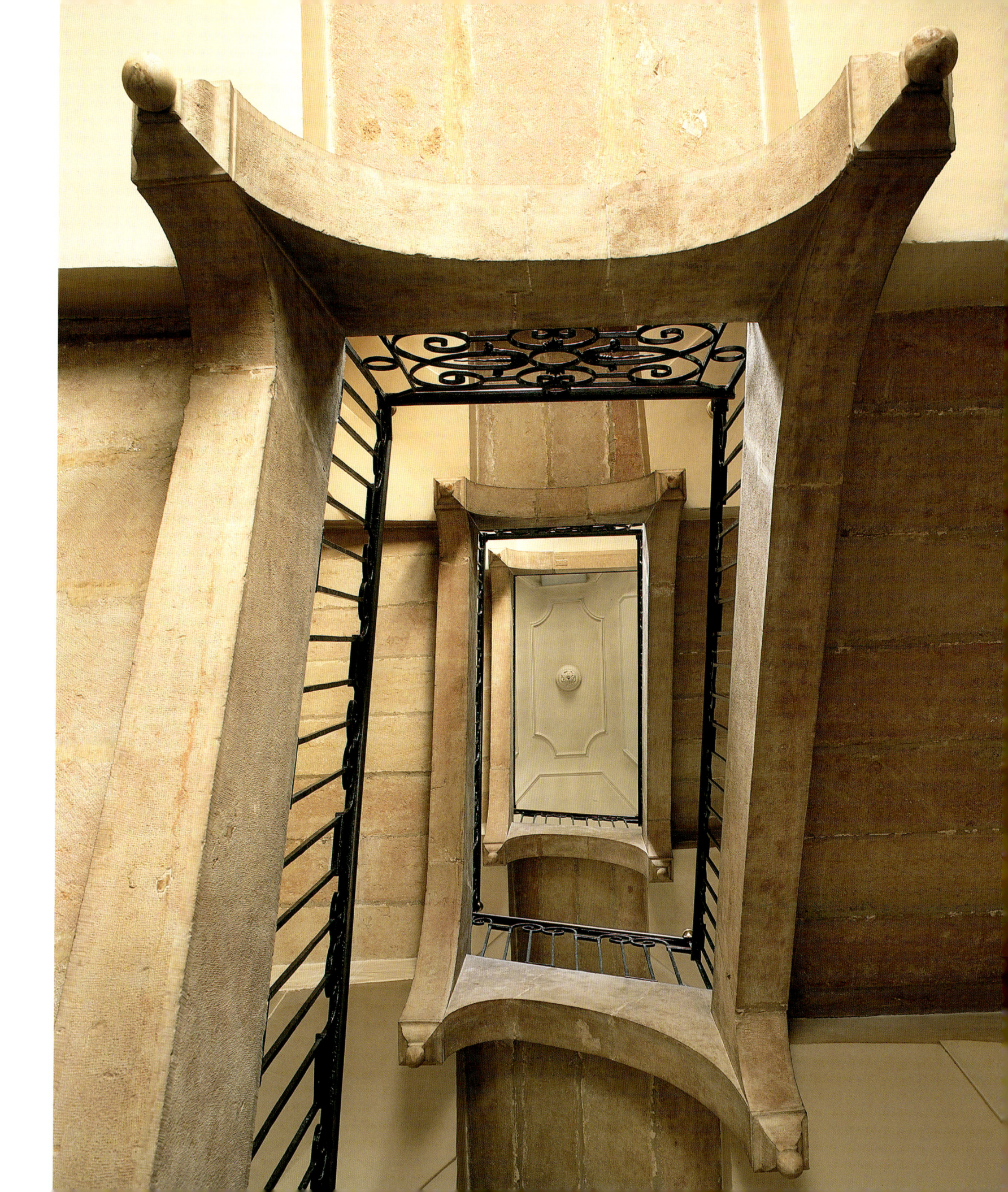

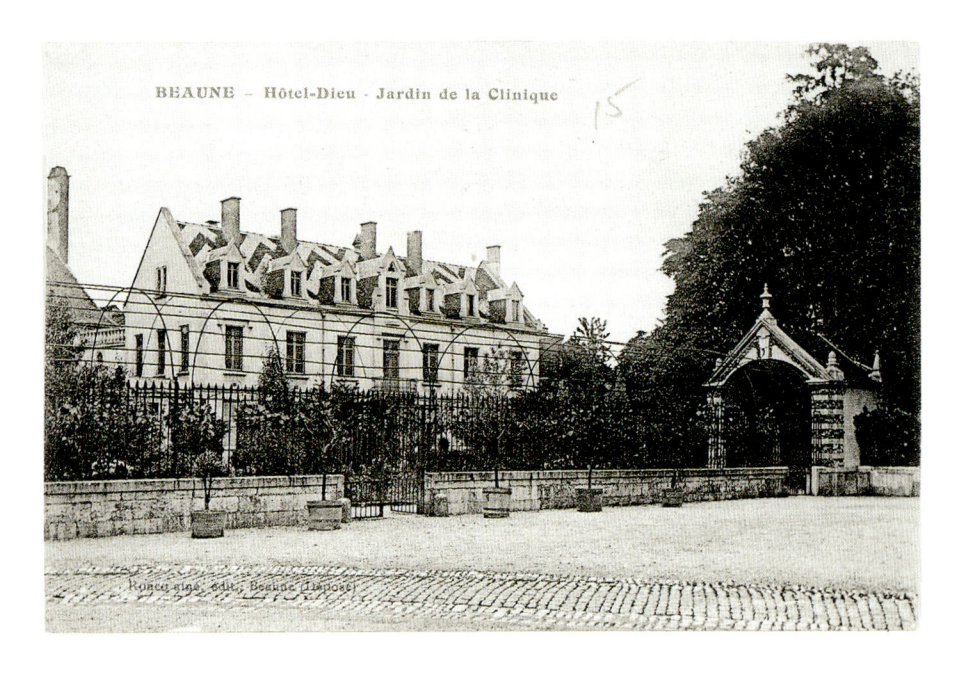

It was closed with the coming of the Revolution and the site later became known as the "woodyard", after a long building used for storing firewood that had been there since the 18th century.

It was here, against the city wall, that six new wards for the mentally ill were built in 1857. Closed off by a wicket-gate, they were small, cold, damp, airless and dark. By 1833 the winepress building was on the point of collapse and had to be demolished – but with great

▌ **Above:** The Bahèzre pavilion, early 20th century.
Right: Quarters for the mentally ill, 19th century.

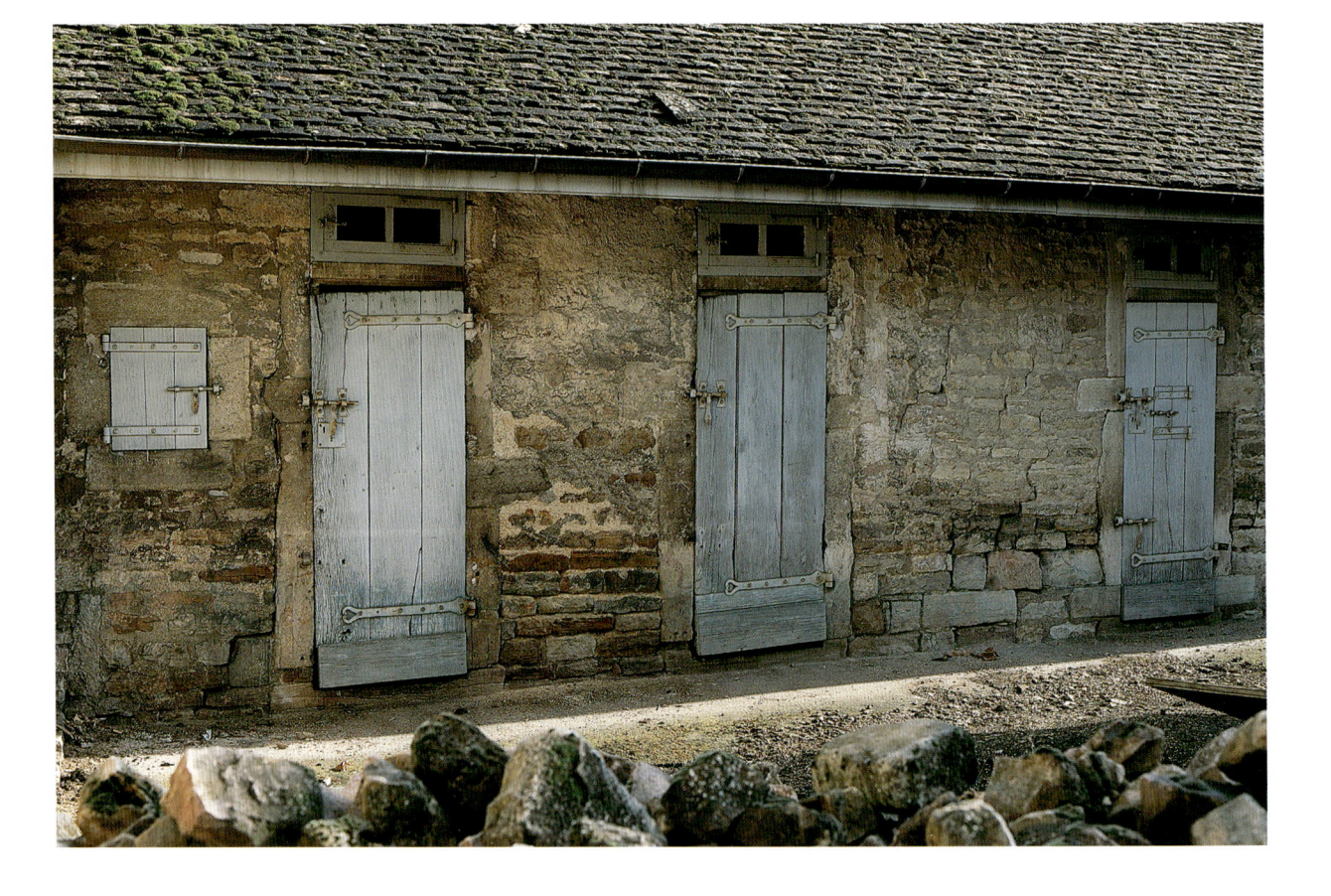

care, for it backed onto a cellar and a barrel-maker's set against the ramparts. It was then rebuilt on the same site, but shortened to allow for a pathway to the gardens and the "woodyard". From the 19th century onwards, and with the exception of the kitchen, the utility rooms were gradually moved out of the medieval hospital compound, firstly to the ground floor of the granary, then to a modest building in the third courtyard, running along the Rue Triperie with the mortuary chapel and the laundry, wash-house and drying room. Ultimately, the decision having been taken to group patients according to illness, new wards had to be created in the rear courtyards. Thus, in 1829-33 the Salle Saint-Joseph – for destitute, incurable patients – was built in the second courtyard, at right angles to the granary, whose façade it imitated.

By 1843 the Hôtel-Dieu had ceased making its own bread, thus rendering the granary superfluous as such. Baths had already been installed in the building early in the 19th century and in 1846 the Salle Sainte-Marguerite and the Salle Parizot were created there. Towards the end of the century Louis Bahèzre de Lanlay bequeathed 170,000 francs for the construction of an operating theatre, laboratory and private rooms: the result was the Neo-Gothic de Bahèzre pavilion, designed by Historical Monuments architect Charles Suisse, who had just rebuilt the spire of the Saint-Bénigne cathedral in Dijon and was also restoring the medieval Château de La Rochepot, not far from Beaune. Radical modernisation and extension of this pavilion have since made it unrecognisable. In 1893-96 the City of Beaune financed the building of a military hospital at the far end of the winepress courtyard, on the site of the "former bursar's office": the Hôtel-Dieu had agreed to relinquish the site in return for the use of the ground floor of the new building. In 1929 the maternity ward, housed in the Salle Parizot since 1896, was transferred there.

In closing, mention should be made of the two oratories built in 1902 in the gardens: they replaced the grottoes of the Nativity and St John, for which there is archival evidence going back to the 18th century.

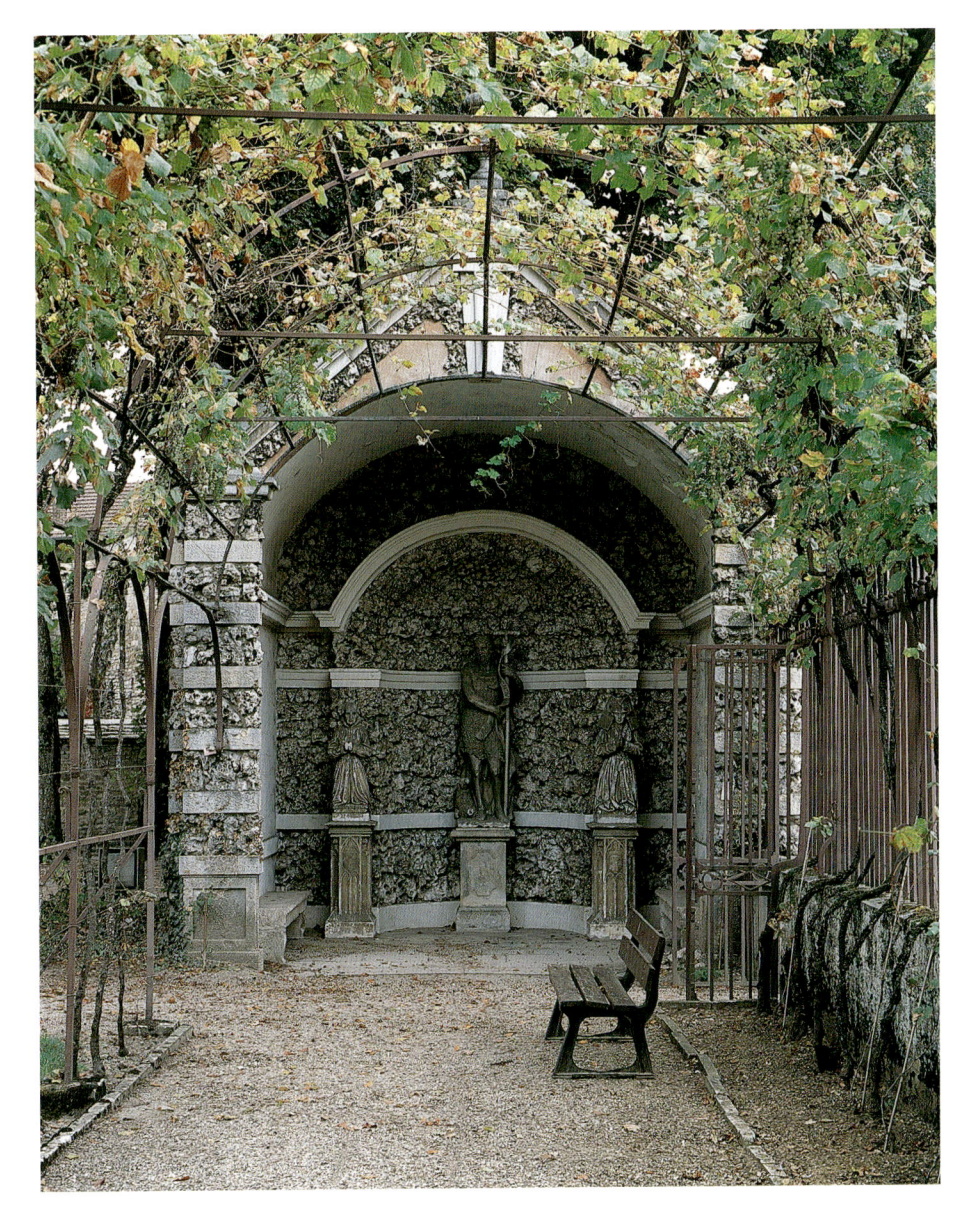

▌ Above: The grotto of St John the Baptist, early 20th century.

Major restoration campaigns

In the 19th century the directors had stated their determination to "recreate Chancellor Rolin's Hôtel-Dieu as it had been when he built it". Already, in anticipation of its four-hundredth anniversary, work carried out in 1841-43 had replaced what time and the Revolution had destroyed, notably the roof ornaments and the Étienne de Saptes statues of the Virgin and Christ on the gables of the main attic. In 1872 the Hôtel-Dieu had paid for the re-rendering of the lower gallery: this brought to light the walled-up medieval doors and windows, which were at once returned to their original function. At the same period Maurice Ouradou had undertaken the restoration of the Great Hall of the Poor. These ventures were the prelude to the large-scale restoration campaigns that began with the 20th century and continue today.

Despite the considerable financial difficulties due to the phylloxera crisis, which cost the establishment a large part of its winemaking-based income, the Hôtel-Dieu, with the assistance of the Education Ministry and the Historical Monuments Department of the time, set about restoring the facades and roofs of the two wings under the supervision of Historical Monuments architect Sauvageot, who brought back the multicoloured roofing. Carried out in 1902-07, these works also involved a return to the wood areas of the first-floor gallery, which had been slated over in the early 19th century and suffered badly in the process, all the protrusions having been cut off. Paris sculptor Adolphe Gleisse provided two little angels to embellish the gables of the two dormer windows over the King's chamber and the former Salle Sainte-Catherine. He also created two plaster models for the gargoyles that Sauvageot added around the upper gallery.

In 1909 Sainte-Anne-Louzier, another Historical Monuments architect, made a proposal for weather-proofing the main building, including the canopy and the spire of the belltower, whose décor of pinnacles and lead-covered false arches he intended to recreate.

▌ Right: One of the angels sculpted by Adolphe Gleisse in the early 20th century.
Facing page: One of the gargoyles designed by Adolphe Gleisse in the early 20th century.

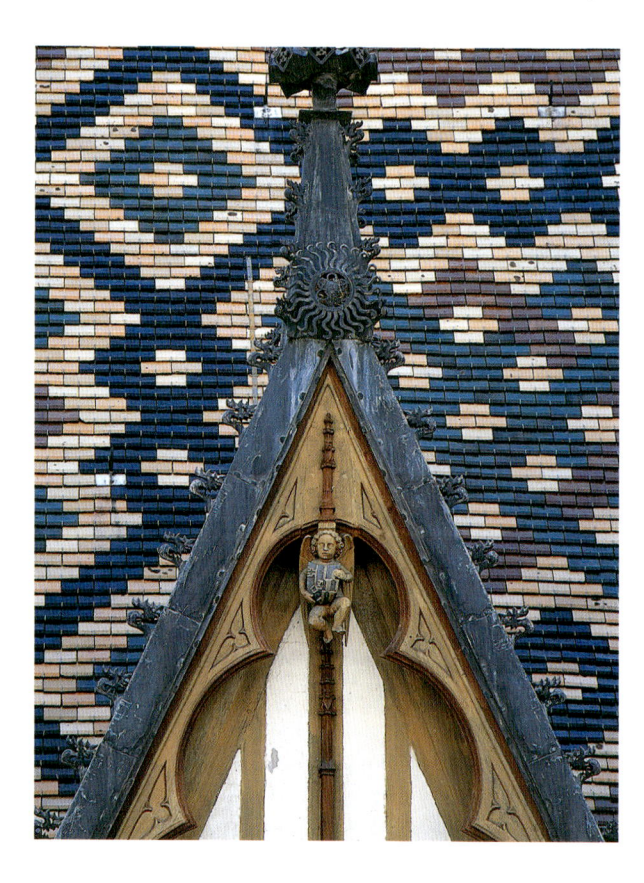

Approval for this controversial project did not come through until 1911, by which time he also wanted to reinstate two vanished rows of "small dormer windows", of which only the rafters bore any trace. For reasons of economy only the lower row was recreated – this seemed to provide adequate ventilation for the attic – and it should be noted that these windows do not appear on the straw model. Sisters Jardeaux et Jacques paid for a new dormer window to light an extension to their dormitory on the courtyard. This long campaign closed in 1937-38 with the restoration of the porch roof.

Work resumed shortly after World War II, with the weatherproofing, the restoration of the lead embellishments and the return of the wood in the upper gallery. The building of a new hospital on another site and the transfer of the patients there in 1971 freed a number of rooms, but the Hôtel-Dieu continued to house the geriatric medicine department. In 1970 the work required by the opening of the building to the public was part of an overall improvements programme, but some decisions were never actually implemented. In 1967 the rear roof-slopes of the two wings giving onto the garden and the Franciscan monastery were restored in line with the Sauvageot model. In 1988-89 Historical Monuments architect Frédéric Didier drew on the straw model for his reroofing of the Salle Saint-Louis with geometrical patterns of glazed tiles. The next step in this process is scheduled for 2007, with restoration of the slate roof of the main attic.

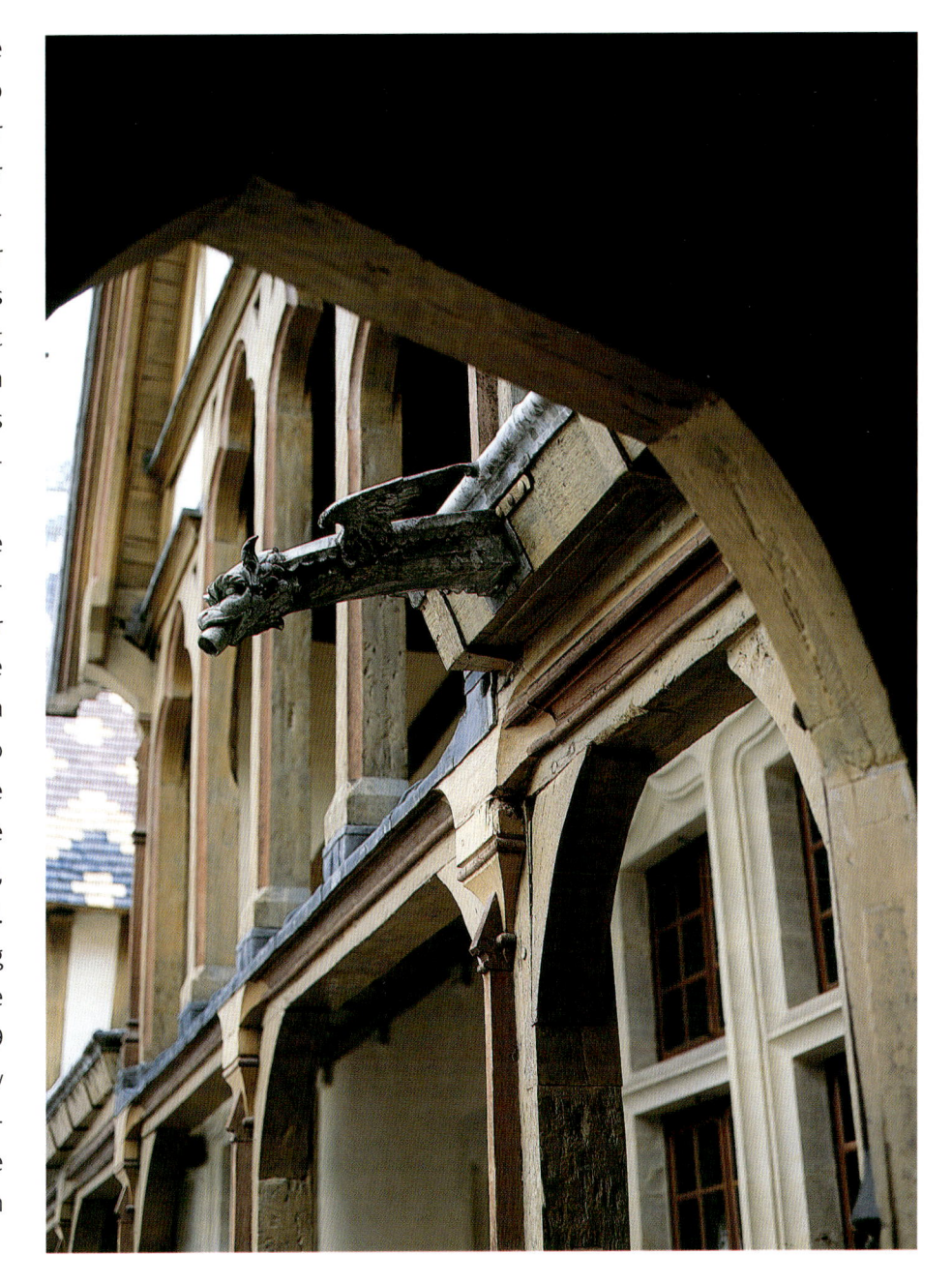

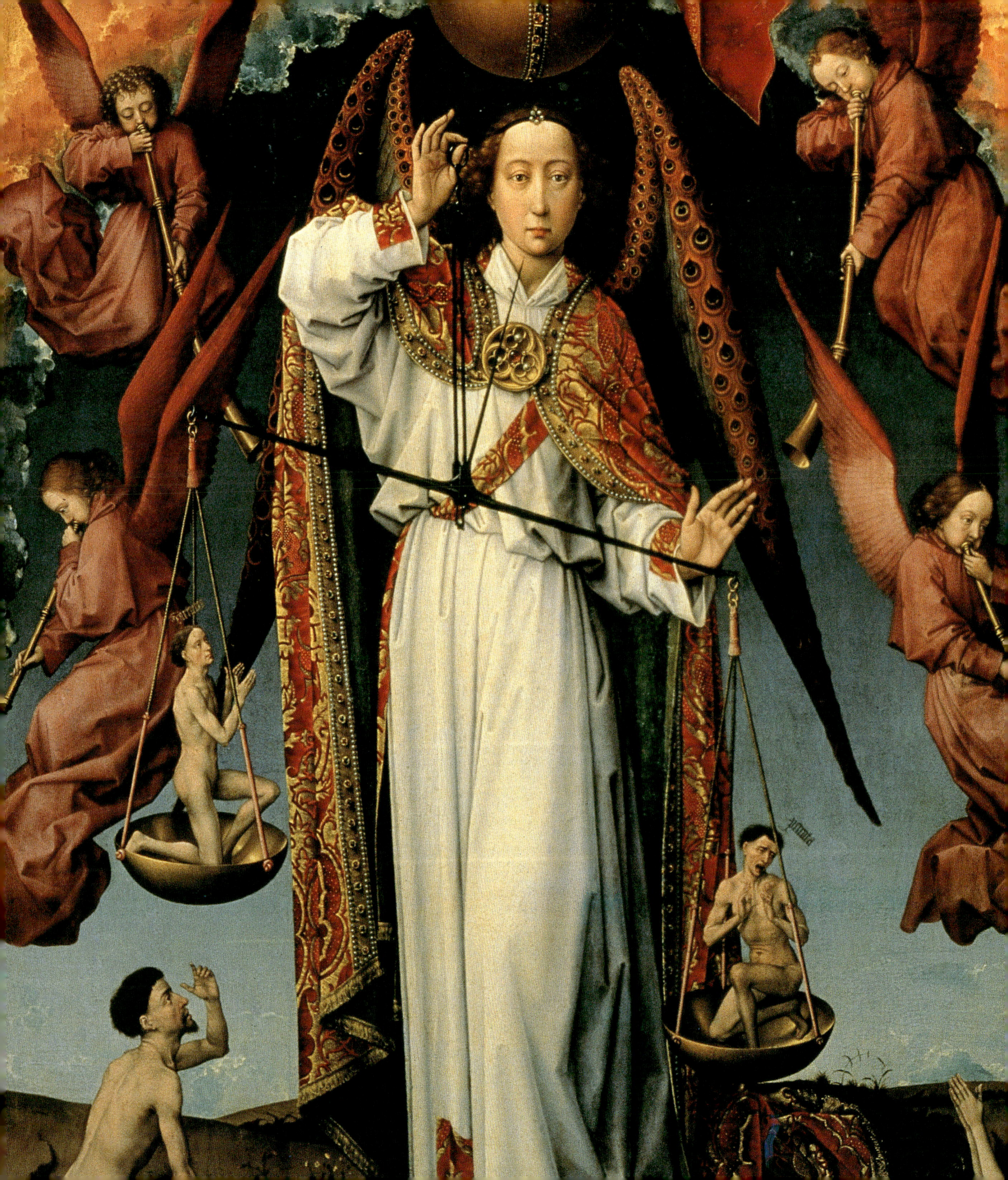

DECORATION AND FURNISHINGS

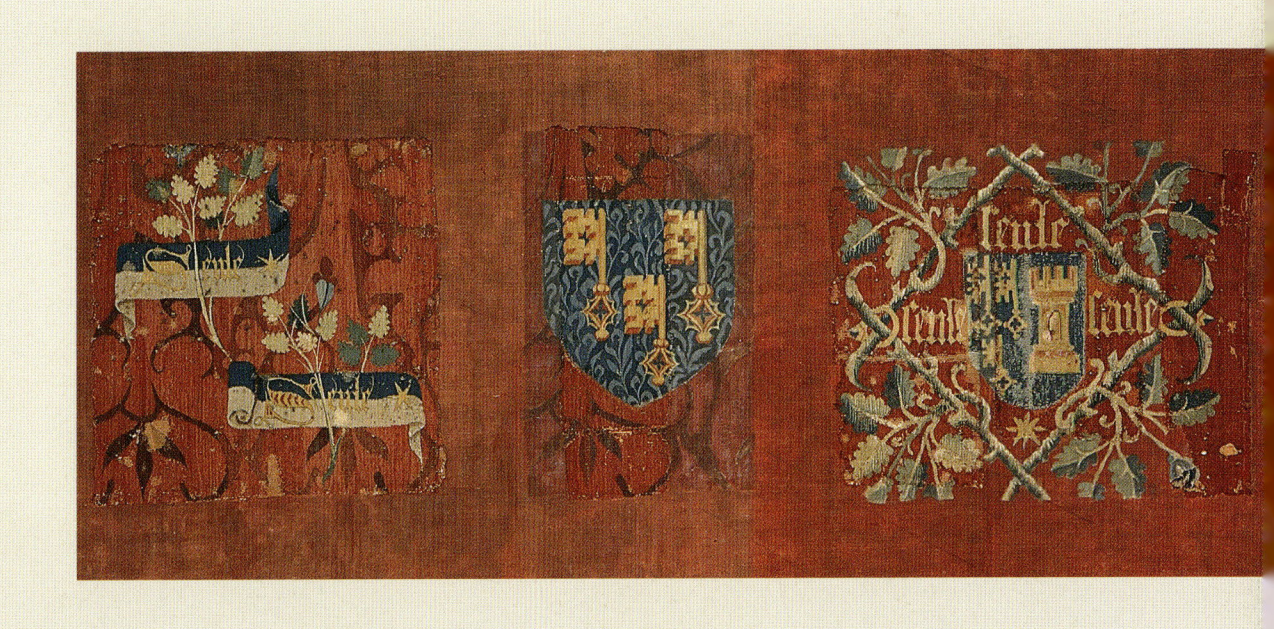

The founders and their image

When he founded the Hôtel-Dieu in Beaune, Nicolas Rolin was one of the richest and most powerful figures of his time. Born into an upper middle-class family in Autun, he embarked on a brilliant career in the service of John the Fearless and Philip the Good, dukes of Burgundy: first a lawyer, then state's counsel, he was appointed chancellor of the dukedom in 1422, matching this political rise with a meteoric social success that saw him knighted in 1424. His plan for founding a hospital took concrete form when he was granted the necessary privileges by Pope Eugene IV in 1441: for a time he hesitated between Beaune and his native Autun, but the nearness of Dijon, capital of the dukedom, and the donation by the City of Beaune of a large area of land doubtless played their part in the final decision.

The underlying intention was dual: Chancellor Rolin wished both to ensure his salvation via works of mercy and to perpetuate his own memory and that of his family. It was not for nothing that, in their own lifetime, he and his wife Guigone de Salins appeared in the Rogier

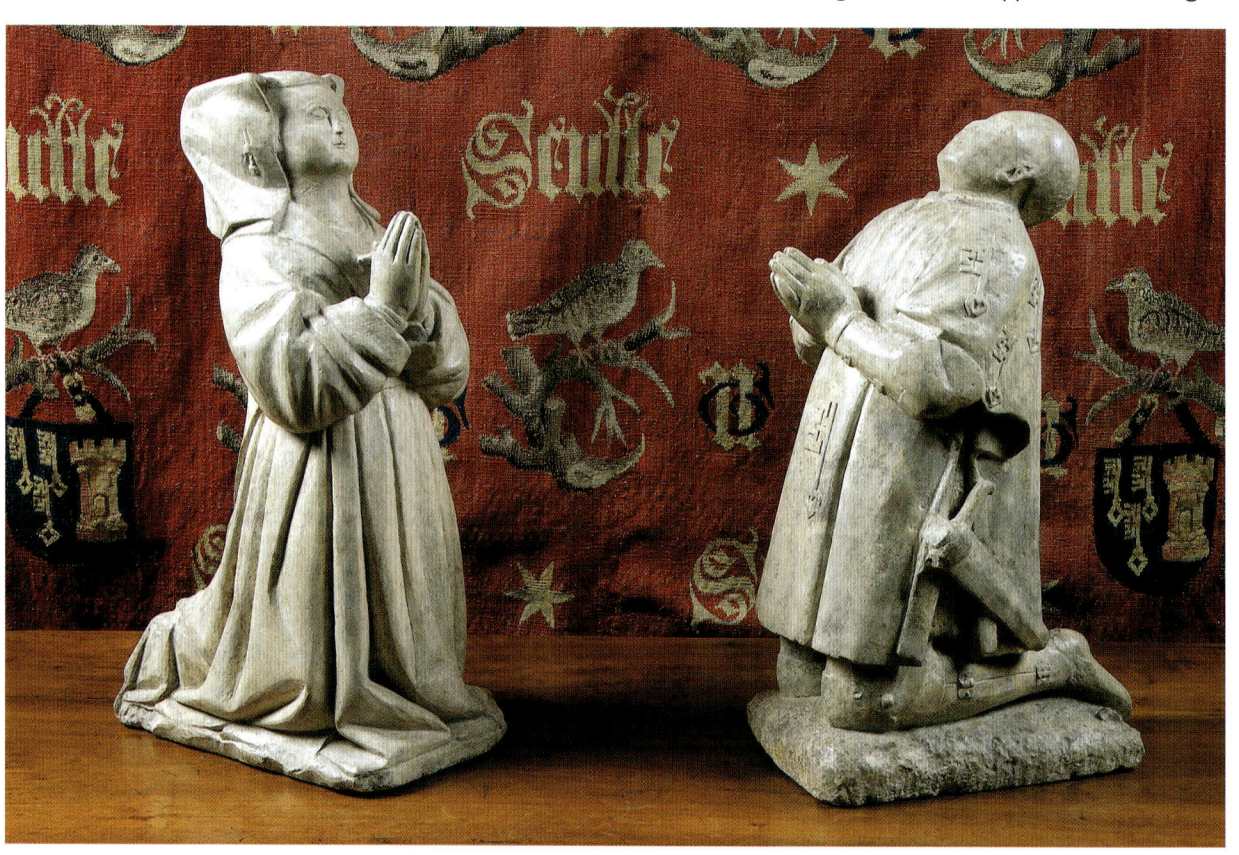

■ Previous pages:
Left: The *Last Judgement* polyptych, by Rogier Van der Weyden (detail).
Right: Fragments of tapestry, mid-15th century.

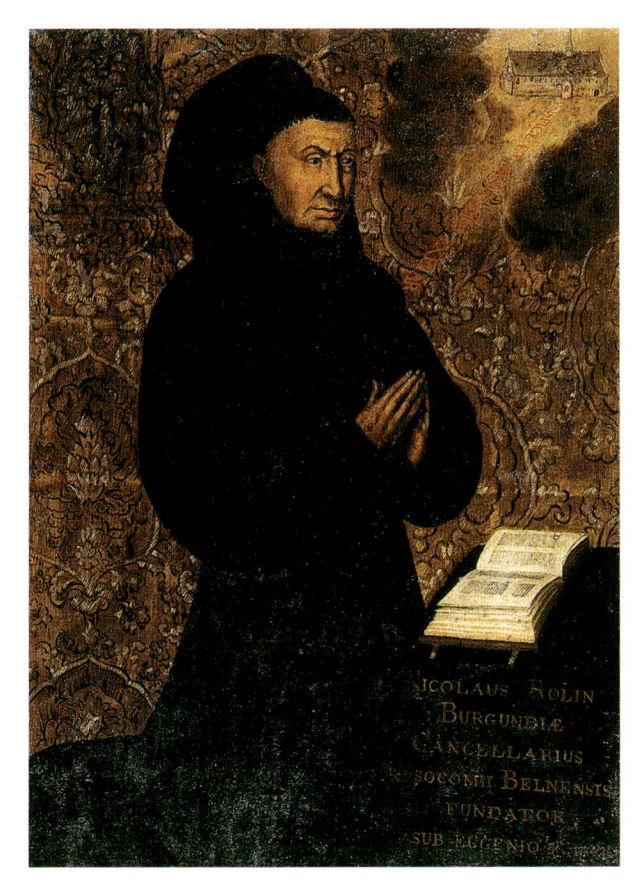

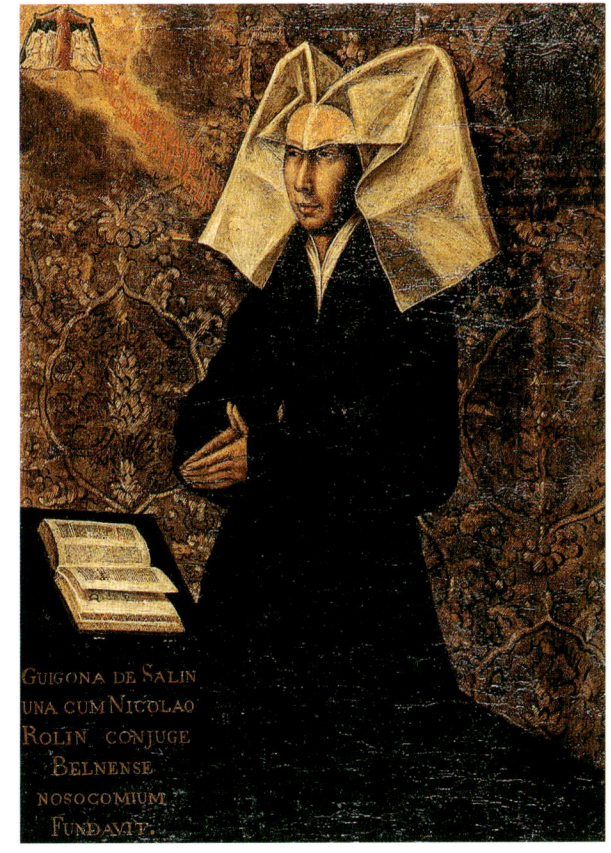

Van der Weyden polyptych and the now lost original stained glass windows of the Hôtel-Dieu chapel. In addition, two contemporary stone statues of the founders, of unknown provenance, are now to be found in the Hospices de Beaune museum. Kneeling with their hands joined, the spouses were doubtless originally set one to each side of a crucified Christ, their faces raised in supplication. Over his armour Nicolas Rolin wears a tabard bearing the three keys of his family coat of arms. Guigone de Salins is dressed in very much the same way as in the polyptych. The faces seem to have been rendered fairly schematically and the degree of wear suggests that the statues had been placed outdoors.

Other images of the founder and his wife created down through the centuries indicate that they were fondly remembered. Two canvases, probably from the 17th century, are adaptations of parts of the *Last Judgement* altarpiece; to one of them the painter has added a view of the Hôtel-Dieu, and to the other Our Lady of Mercy sheltering the hospitaller nuns under her cloak.

The 19th century saw two stained glass portrayals of the founders succeed each other in the central window of the Great Hall of the Poor. The 1844 version by Clermont-Ferrand glassmaker Étienne Thevenot shows them accompanied by St Nicholas and St Anthony, the latter – the Hôtel-Dieu's principal patron saint – being especially venerated by Guigone. In 1877 the painter-glassmaker Louis Ottin restored the imagery of this window to match a description dating from 1653: here we find the founders again, with Philip the Good and Isabelle of Portugal, in a scene including a Crucifixion and Our Lady of Mercy.

In 1844 the Brotherhood of the Holy Spirit commissioned Étienne de Saptes to sculpt two portraits of the founders for the chapel choir. These statues are now in a rocaille oratory at the bottom of the garden.

The Burgundy-born sculptor Henri Bouchard returned to the subject in 1912, with models for two full-size standing statues. With slight modifications these were executed in stone and placed in the second courtyard in 1921 and 1923.

▌ Facing page: Donor statues, mid-15th century. Above: Portraits of the founders: oil on canvas, 17th century.

Caring for the soul

In the philosophy of the medieval hospital the salvation of the soul was inseparable from the health of the body. This concern with providing patients with spiritual consolation and ensuring eternal happiness for the dying is manifest in the presence of an altar for celebrating mass in every ward and of devotional paintings and statues as sources of courage and hope.

ROGIER VAN DER WEYDEN'S MASTERPIECE

The chapel's handsomest ornament was the *Last Judgement* reredos, formerly set over the marble altar and now preserved in a specially air-conditioned room. Originally comprising nine oak panels, six of them painted on both sides, this polyptych is the largest of Van der Weyden's altarpieces and the pinnacle of his mature period. It was also Nicolas Rolin's major donation to the hospital he founded. No documentary evidence concerning the work's commissioning has been found, but it seems likely that it was already in place when the chapel was consecrated on 31 December 1451; thus its creation would date from the period between 1443 – the foundation year – and 1451.

It is no coincidence that the chancellor called in the official painter of the City of Brussels, for he often spent time there with the duke's court. This use of a highly respected Flemish painter also points up an urge to affirm the social status that came with recent ennoblement. Portrayed, with his wife Guigone de Salins, as a donor on the back of the end panels – now on show separately – Nicolas Rolin asserts his lordly rank with his coat of arms on a shield topped with a helmet, and with the tapestry, also bearing the coat of arms, draped over the prie-dieu. Dressed in black – a fashion established by Philip the Good – the spouses pray before *grisaille* trompe-l'œil statues of St Sebastian and St Anthony, whom they both venerated and who were frequently invoked in times of plague. Above, in the same monochrome style, is the scene of the Annunciation.

In contrast with this soberness of tone, the front of the reredos is a riot of colour dominated by red and by the gold of the background. Here chromatic richness and beauty are the driving force for a clear-cut, hierarchical composition dominated by the heavenly court and curiously free of any demonic presence. The focal point is the central panel, dominated by the majestic figure of the resurrected Christ wearing a scarlet cloak and enthroned on a rainbow; his feet rest on a globe of the world and his wounds suggest rubies. To each side angels in white hold up the instruments of his passion. Like Christ himself, the heavenly court is set against a gold background edged with scarlet clouds – an evocation of eternal light. In the foreground the Virgin Mary and St John the Baptist intercede with the Supreme Judge, while behind them the apostles sit in a semi-circle with saints.

▌ Facing page: Rear view of the *Last Judgment* polyptych, painted by Rogier Van der Weyden, mid-15th century.

69

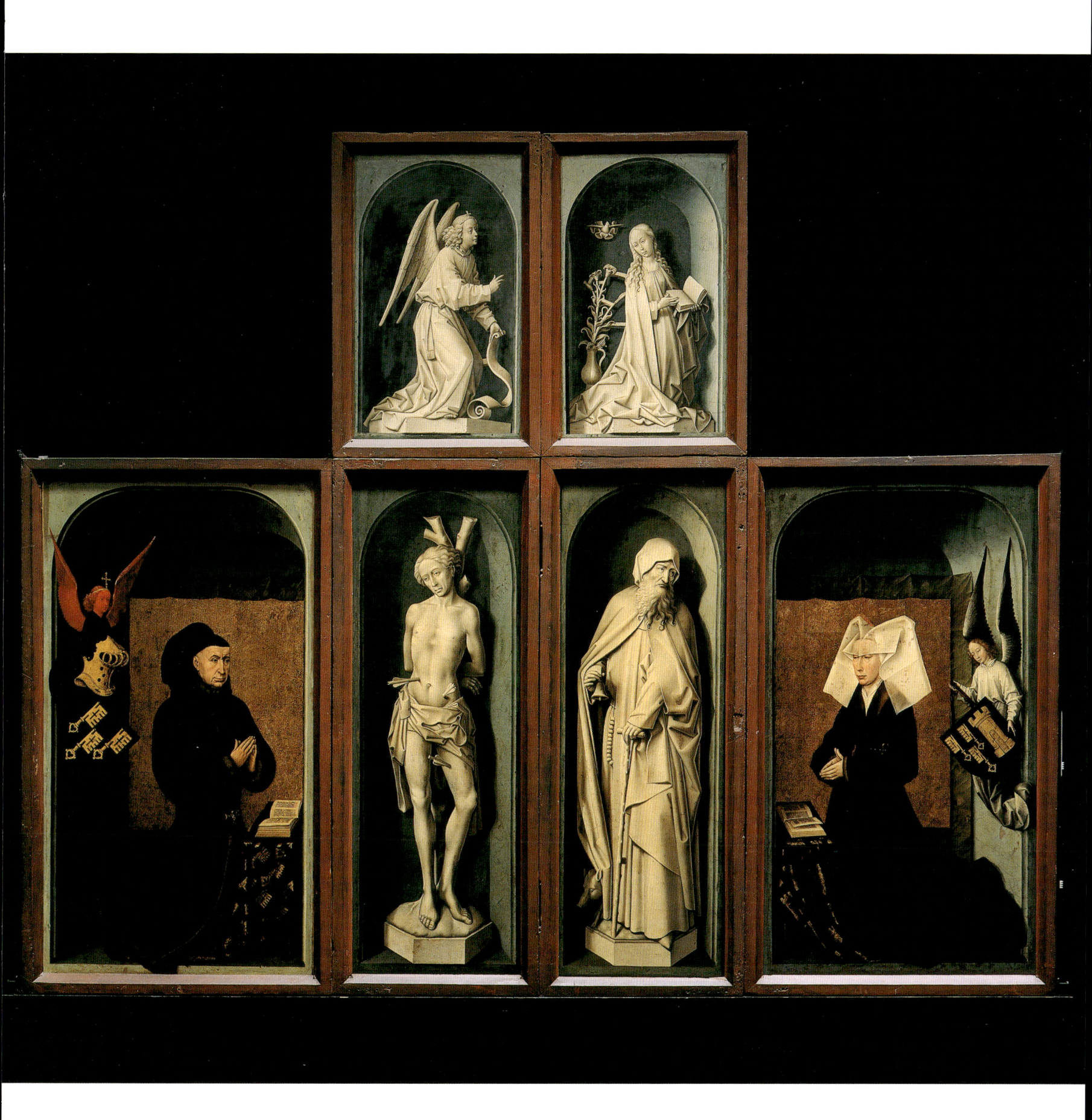

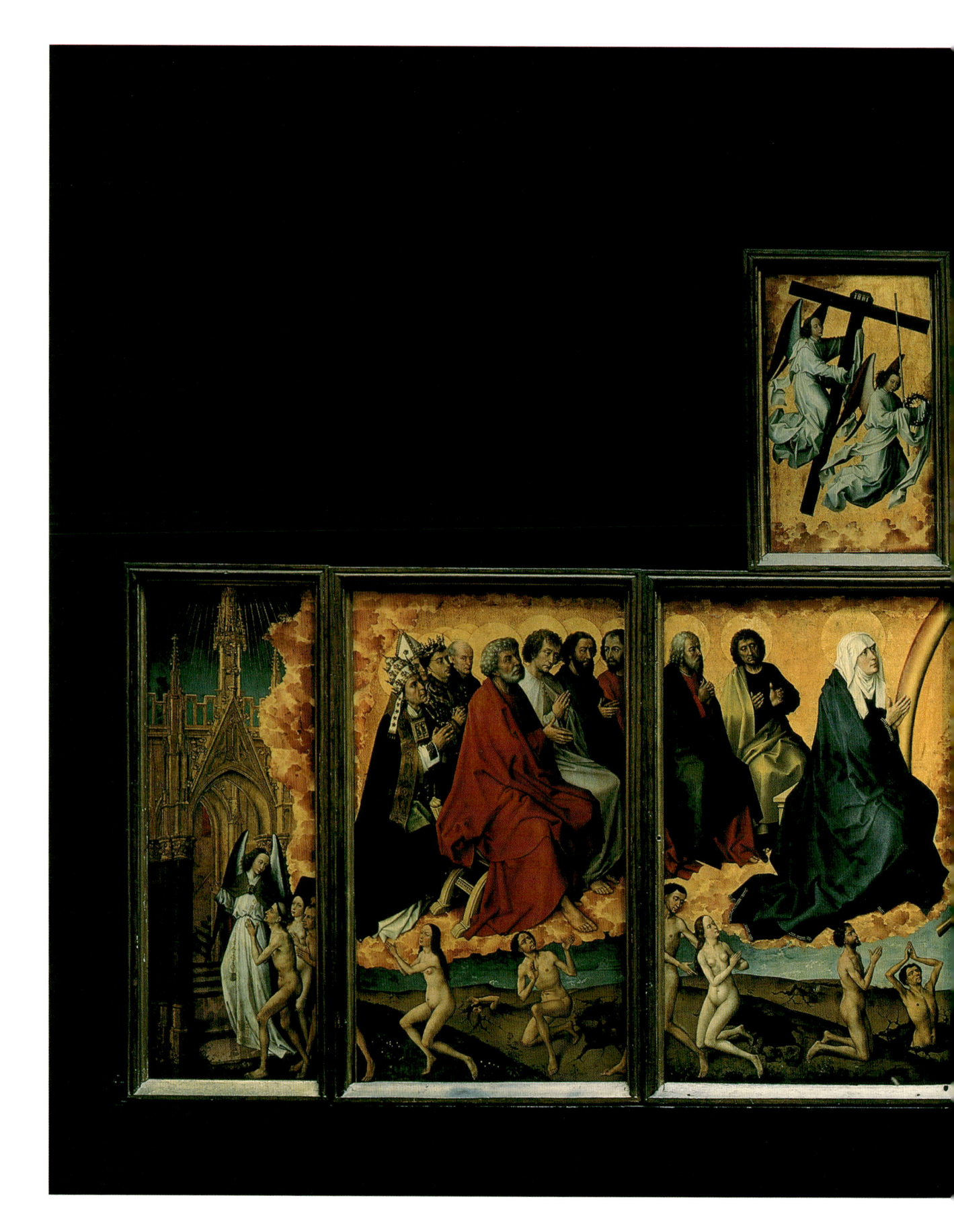

The *Last Judgment* polyptych by Rogier Van der Weyden, mid-15th century.

71

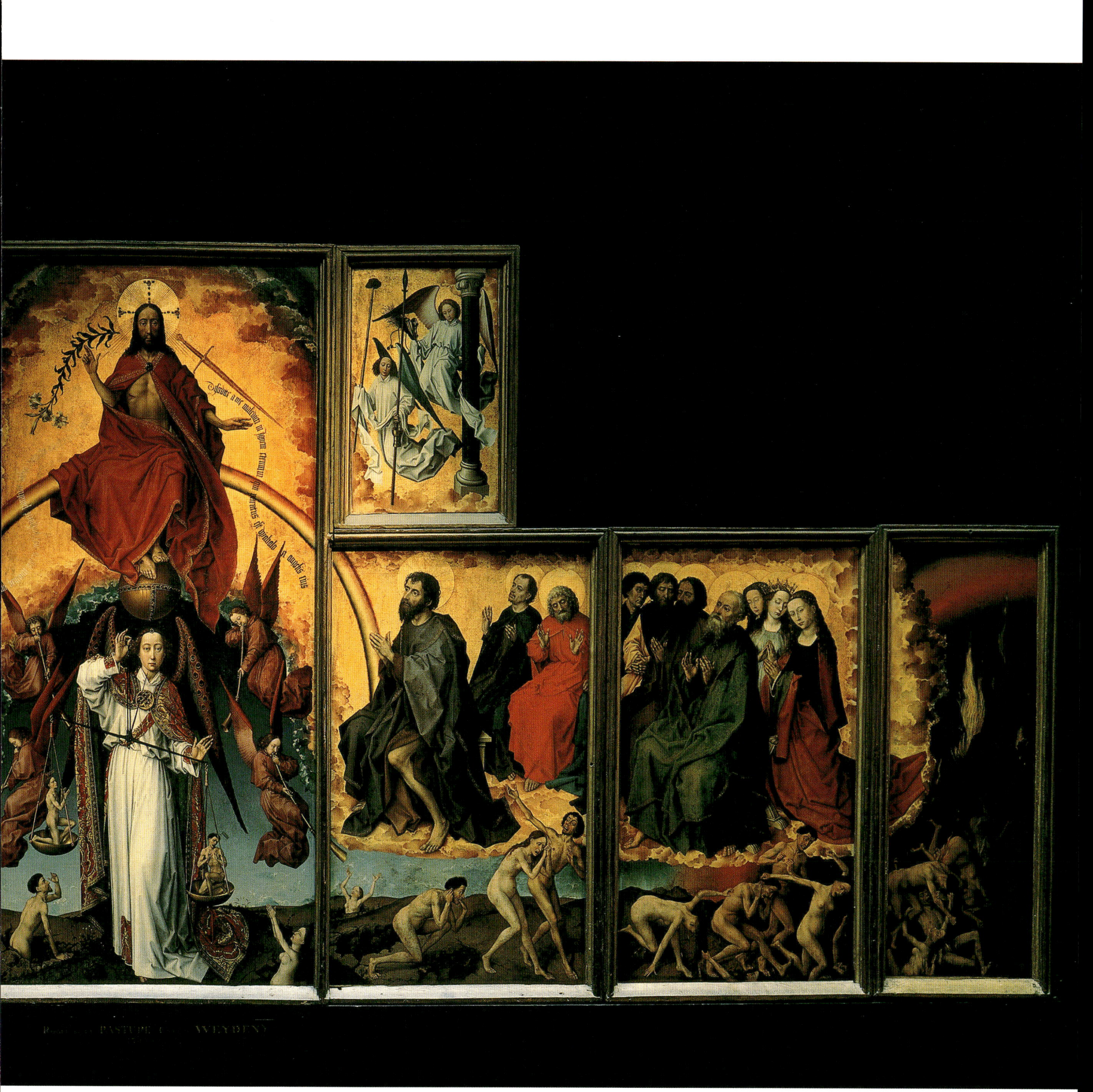

Directly below in the same panel a highly innovative parallel has the archangel Michael, clad in an alb and a brocade cope, adopting the same pose as Christ. Flanked by four angels calling the dead to judgment with trumpets, Michael holds a scales, each of whose trays bears a tiny figure: the higher one symbolises virtue, while on the other side sin pulls the beam downwards. At the archangel's feet the dead rise up out of the earth: to his left the damned, bent and grimacing, traverse cracked and broken ground in their headlong flight into the burning depths of hell, while to his right the chosen, erect, cross a field of flowers towards the golden gates.

Perfectly suited to a hospital, where questions of life, death and the beyond take on a special poignancy, this Last Judgement portrays Christ's triumph over death, the promise of the beatific vision, and the notion of that ultimate judgement as hinging on works of mercy.

Created specifically for the Hôtel-Dieu, the polyptych has rarely ventured elsewhere, although a notable absence was its departure to the Louvre workshops for restoration in 1875-78. It has been a classified Historical Monument since 1891.

TAPESTRIES AND TEXTILES IN THE CHAPELS

Guigone de Salins is given no mention in the Hôtel-Dieu's founding declaration, but it is clear that she felt great affection for the hospital to which she retired after the death of her husband in 1462 and where she was buried in 1470. Her cherished project was the decoration of the chapel, where four tapestries bear her coat of arms.

Two of the tapestries show St Anthony, the Hôtel-Dieu's principal patron saint, against a backdrop of doves matching that on the woven bed covers in the Great Hall. On feast days these tapestries were laid on the seats of the celebrants near the high altar.

The focal point of the other two is the blood of the Lamb – the symbol of Jesus – flowing into a chalice. The blue background alternates the keys and the tower to be found, respectively, on the Rolin and Salins coats of arms. The larger one decorated the pulpit, the smaller one the front of the altar.

The antependium or frontal – the hanging on the altar-front – was changed according to the liturgical feast days. Each of the altars in the hospital wards had several antependia.

The Annunciation hanging, made for the altar in the Salle Notre-Dame, has a blue velvet background sprinkled with stars and overlaid with the figures of the Virgin and the angel Gabriel in multicoloured embroidered silk appliqué stitched with gold and silver. This piece dates from the founding era, tradition having it that it was embroidered by Guigone de Salins when she was widowed.

The 1501 inventory makes mention of another 15th-century work, "a large altar frontal of painted cloth showing Christ in majesty and the four evangelists".

■ Facing page, top: *St Anthony*, tapestry, 1443-62. Listed as a historical monument in 1943.
Facing page, bottom: *The Blood of the Lamb*, tapestry 1462-70. Listed as a historical monument in 1943.

73

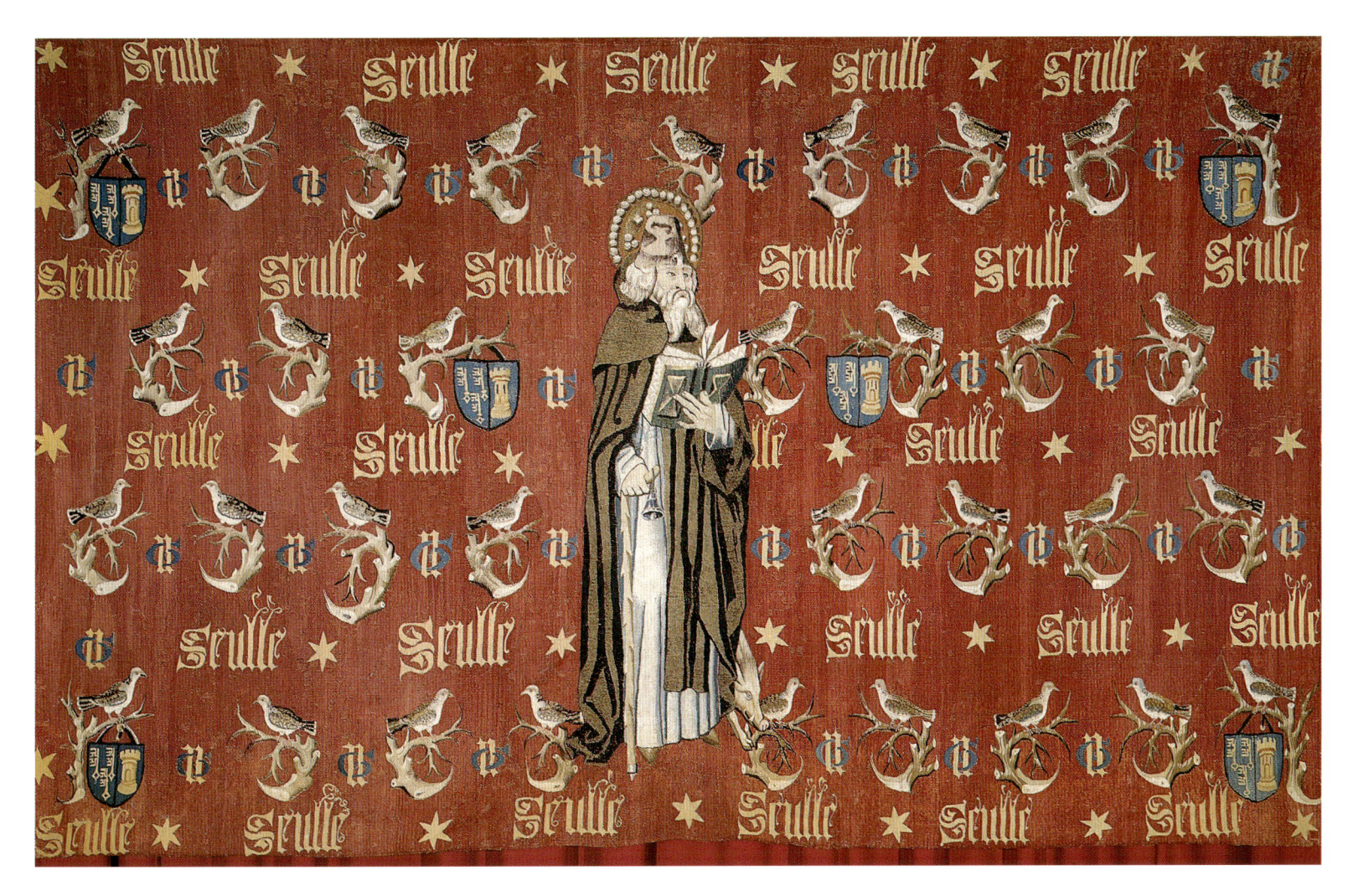

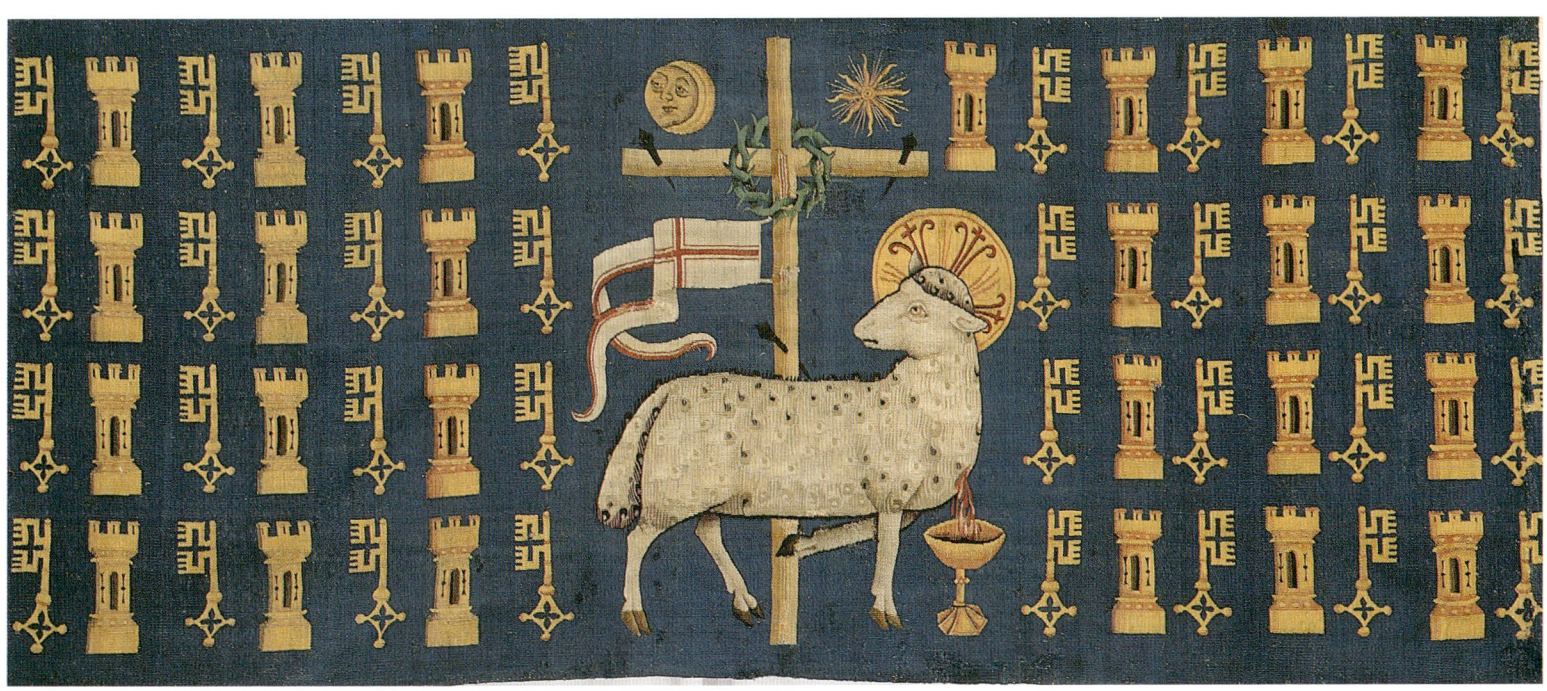

74

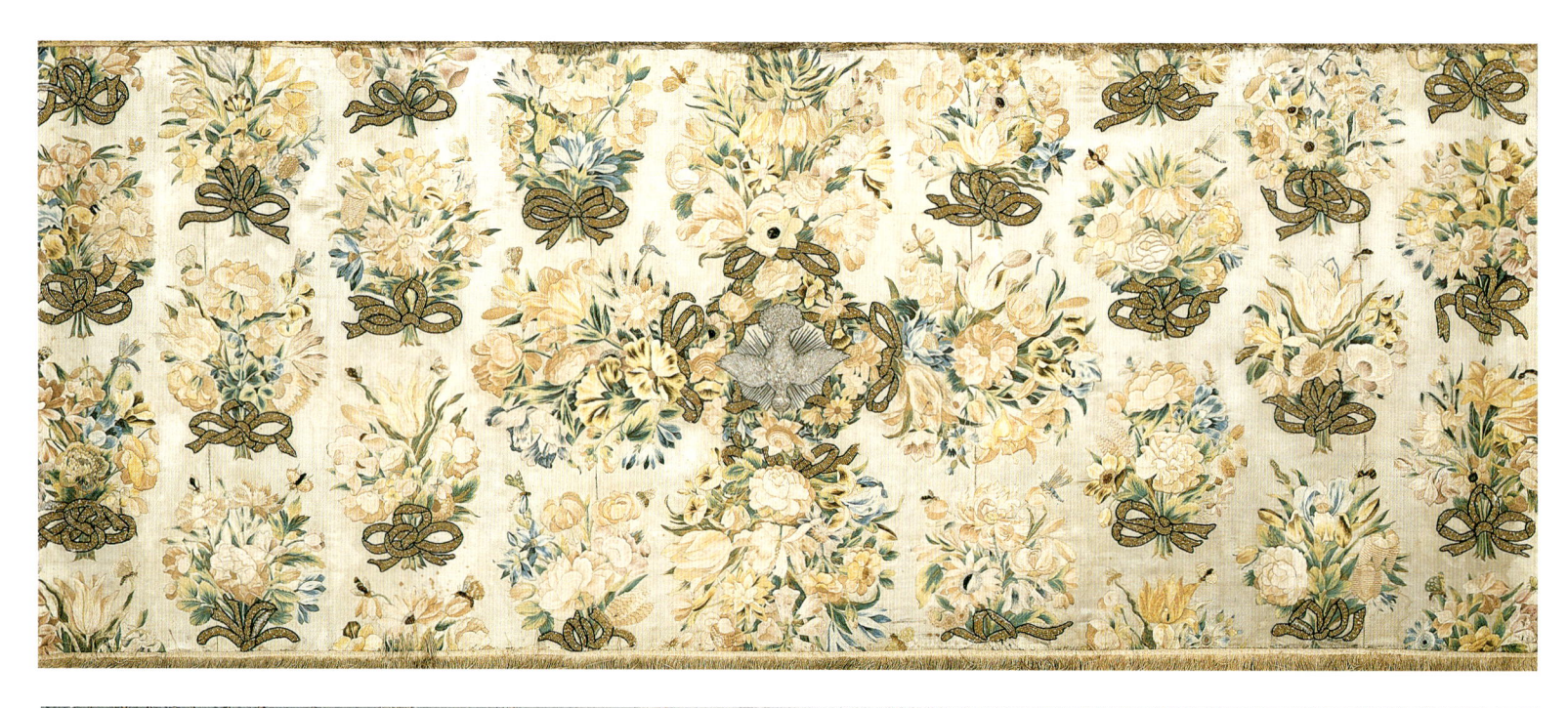

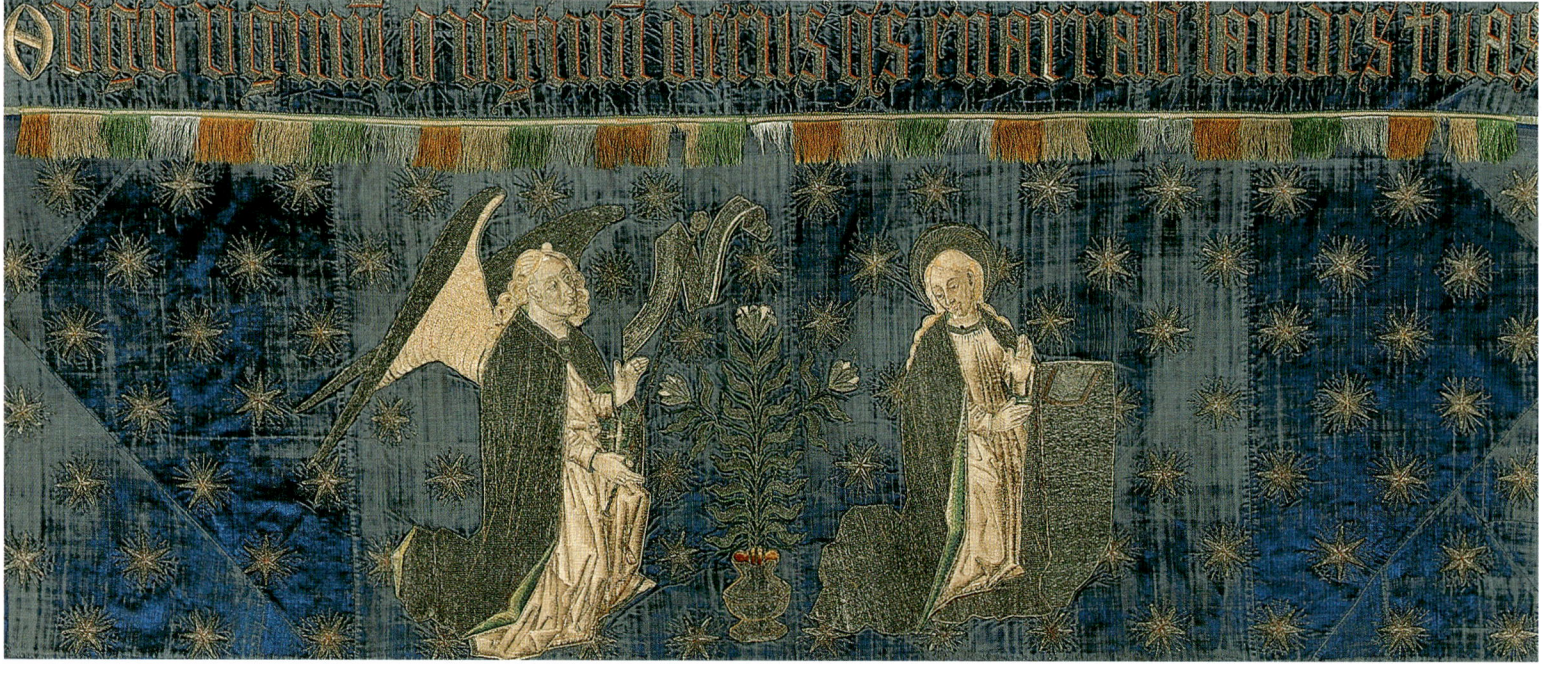

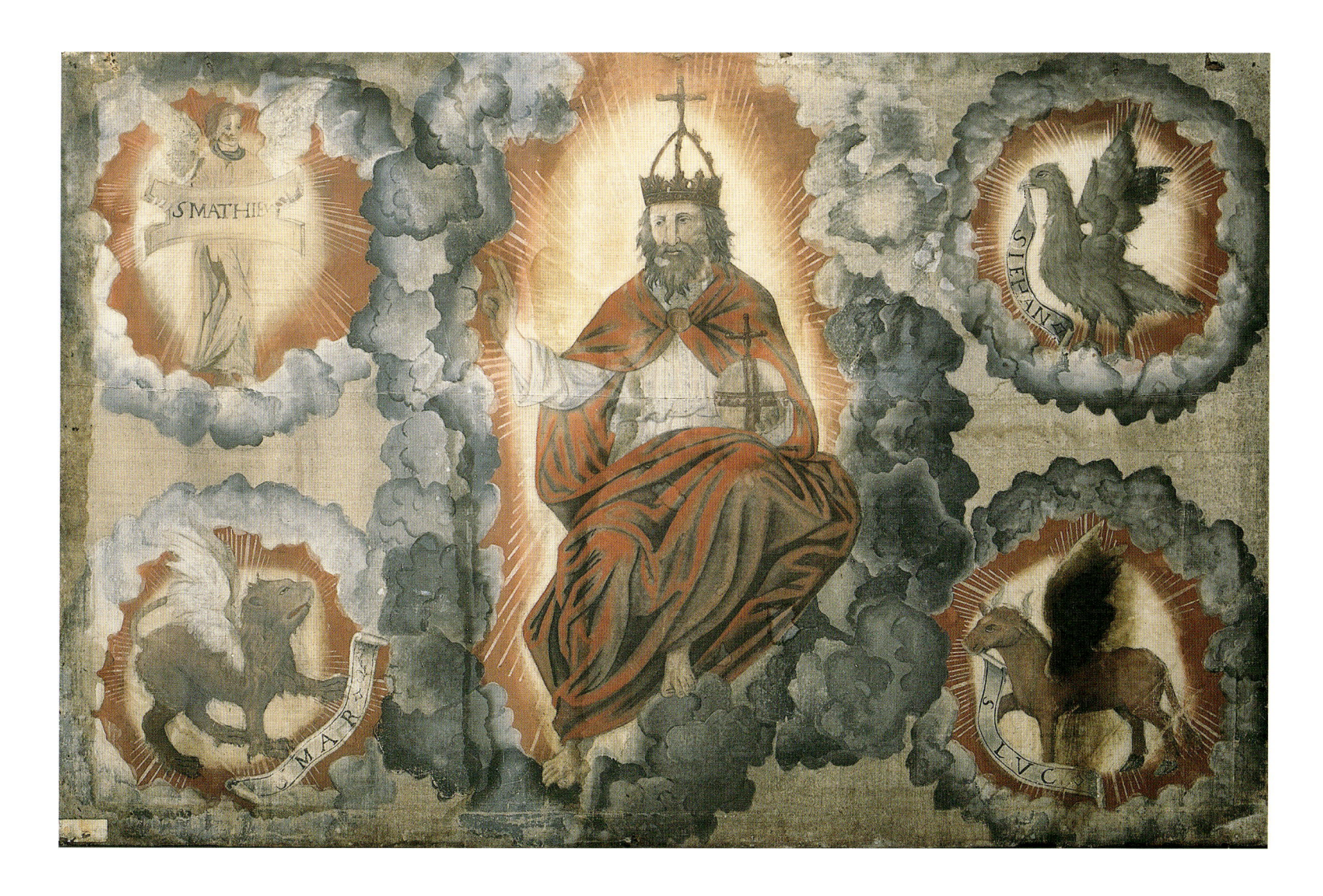

This distemper painting on linen in fact portrays Christ surrounded by symbols of the evangelists – the angel of Matthew, the eagle of John, the lion of Mark and the bull of Luke – and shining forth amid the heavenly hosts. Their extreme fragility has meant that very few paintings of this kind have come down to us.

In a very different decorative style, the frontal of the altar of the Holy Spirit was created in the 18th century by nuns from Beaune – perhaps Carmelites, highly reputed for their embroidery skills. The grey-beige satin, embroidered with multicoloured silk and white and gold glass beads, is dotted with bouquets linked by a ribbon and swarming with various insects. At the centre four of them form a cross around the dove of the Holy Spirit.

THE PAINTINGS

Borne in Beaune, Hugues Bétauld was "receveur des consignations" at the Parliament in Paris, and personally financed the building and decoration of a new ward, the Salle Saint-Hugues. Chosen to carry out the decoration was Isaac Moillon (1614-1673), court painter in 1655 and admitted to the Royal Academy in 1663.

His work on the walls includes nine *Miracles of Christ*, each in a trompe-l'œil frame under which a verse text explains the scene. Determinedly monumental, the paintings are typical of the sweeping, somewhat heavyhanded style Moillon often resorted to in the course of his career. His miraculous cures and resurrections were doubtless intended as messages of

▌Facing page, top:
The antependium – the frontal altar hanging – of the *Annunciation*, second half 15th century. Listed as a historical monument in 1944.
Facing page, bottom:
Altar cloth, 18th century
Above: *Christ and the Tetramorph*,
late 15th century.

76

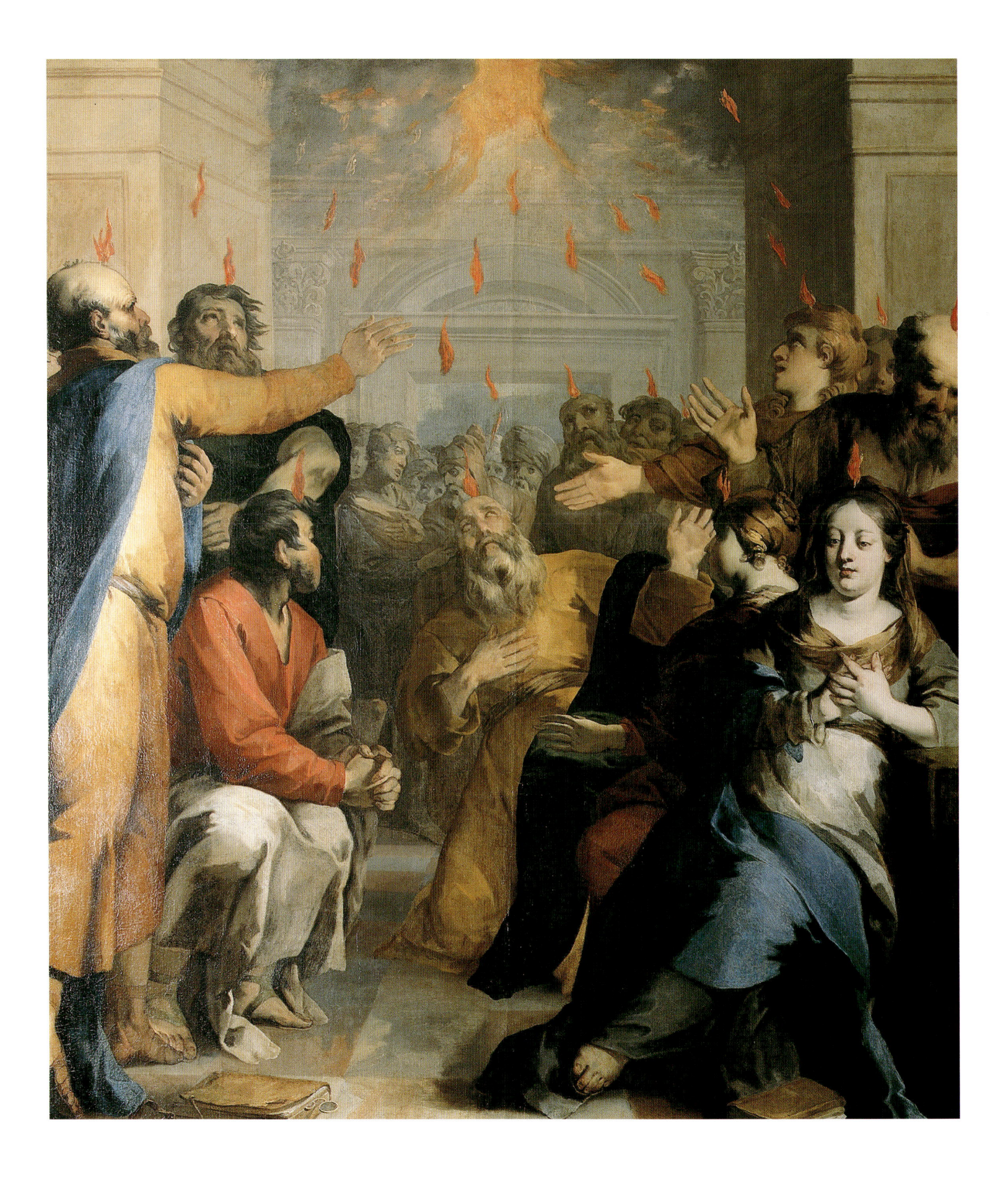

77

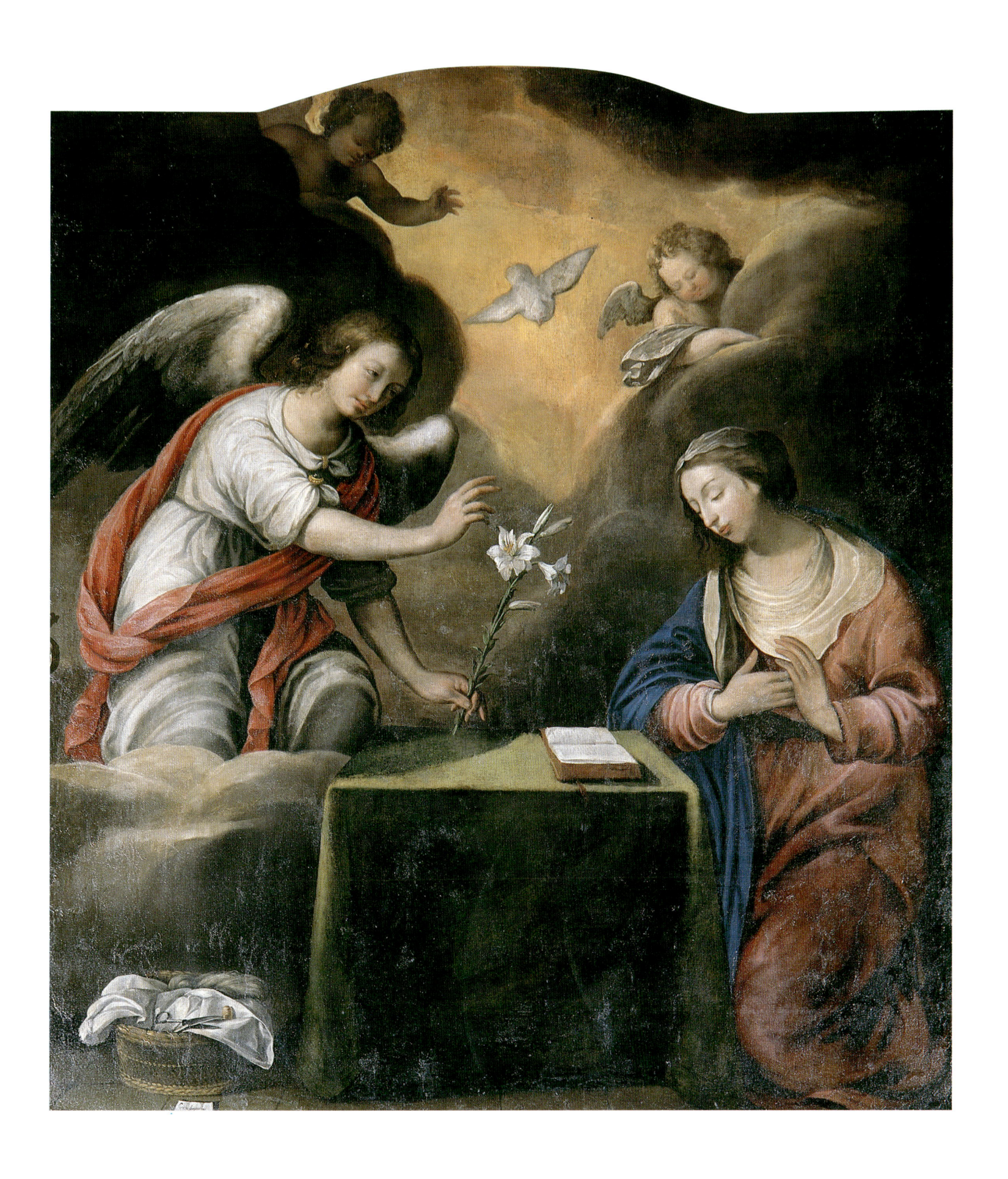

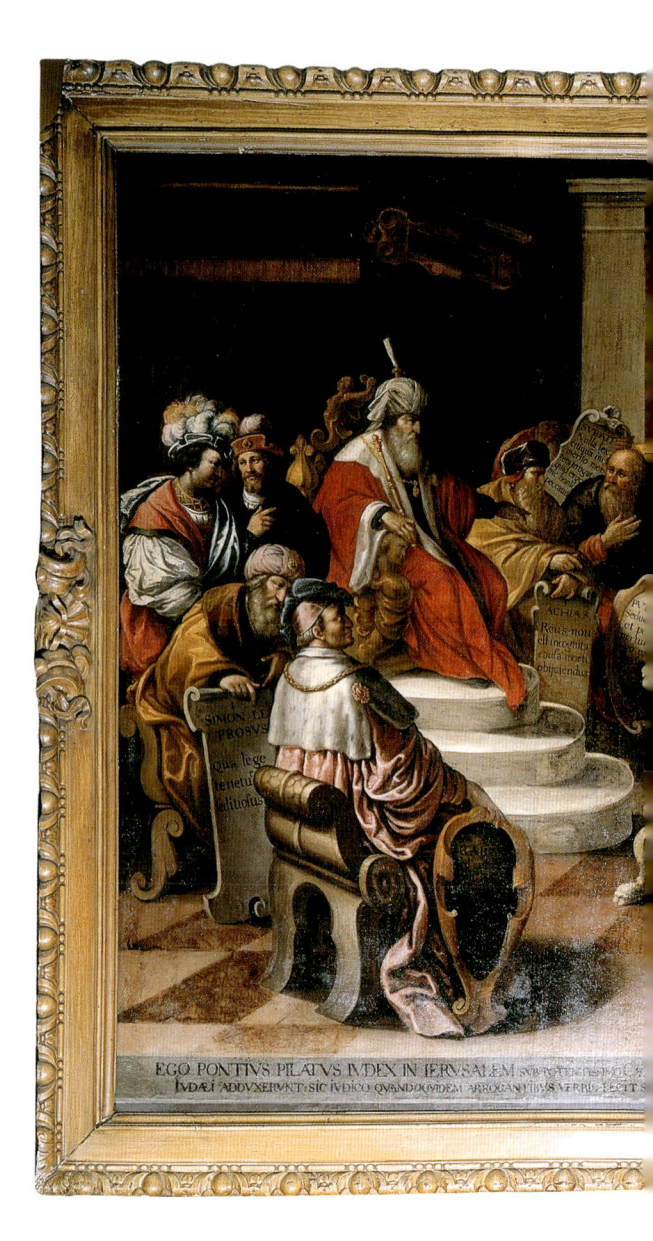

hope for the patients, probably uneducated people to whom this unsubtle approach was well suited. The ceiling is decorated with a large Mannerist canvas, signed and dated 1646 and showing Jesus curing a cripple at the pool of Bethesda. Here the artist has disregarded the rules of his time, which held it inappropriate to show "water on the ceiling", as the viewer would have the feeling of being at the bottom of a pool. When it was restored in 1946, the canvas was cut into forty rectangular panels and marouflaged on hardboard.

Above the altar in this ward can be seen the *Miracle of St Hugh*, in which the painter seems to have combined two scenes via a procedure that was already archaic by the 17th century: shown drowned in the foreground, the child is then seen resuscitated, with his mother. The scale and chromatic harmony of the work illustrate the undeniable gifts of the artist. The image is flanked by angels painted in monochrome on wood.

In Guigone de Salins' room Moillon used warm tones for his *Pentecost*, notable for its off-centre positioning of the Virgin: she was usually placed in the midst of the apostles, as is the case in another treatment of the same subject, a copy of a work by the Italian painter Vasari, in the Salle Saint-Nicolas.

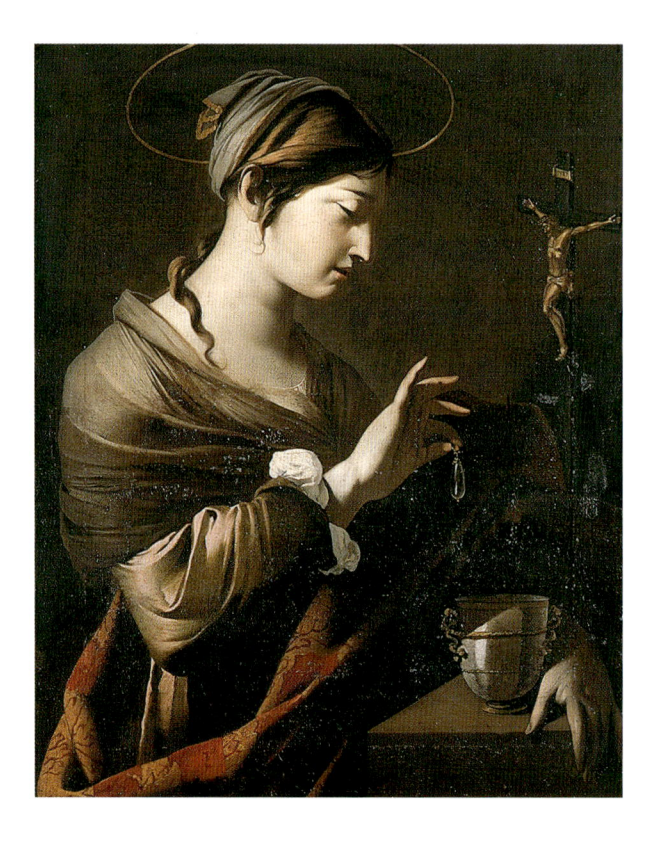

■ Previous pages:
Left: *Pentecost* by Isaac Moillon.
Right: *The Annunciation* by Luc Despesches, first half 17th century, listed as a historical monument in 1971
Right: *St Pelagia* by Jean Tassel, first half 17th century.
Above right: *Christ before Caiaphas*, oil on canvas dated 1641.

78

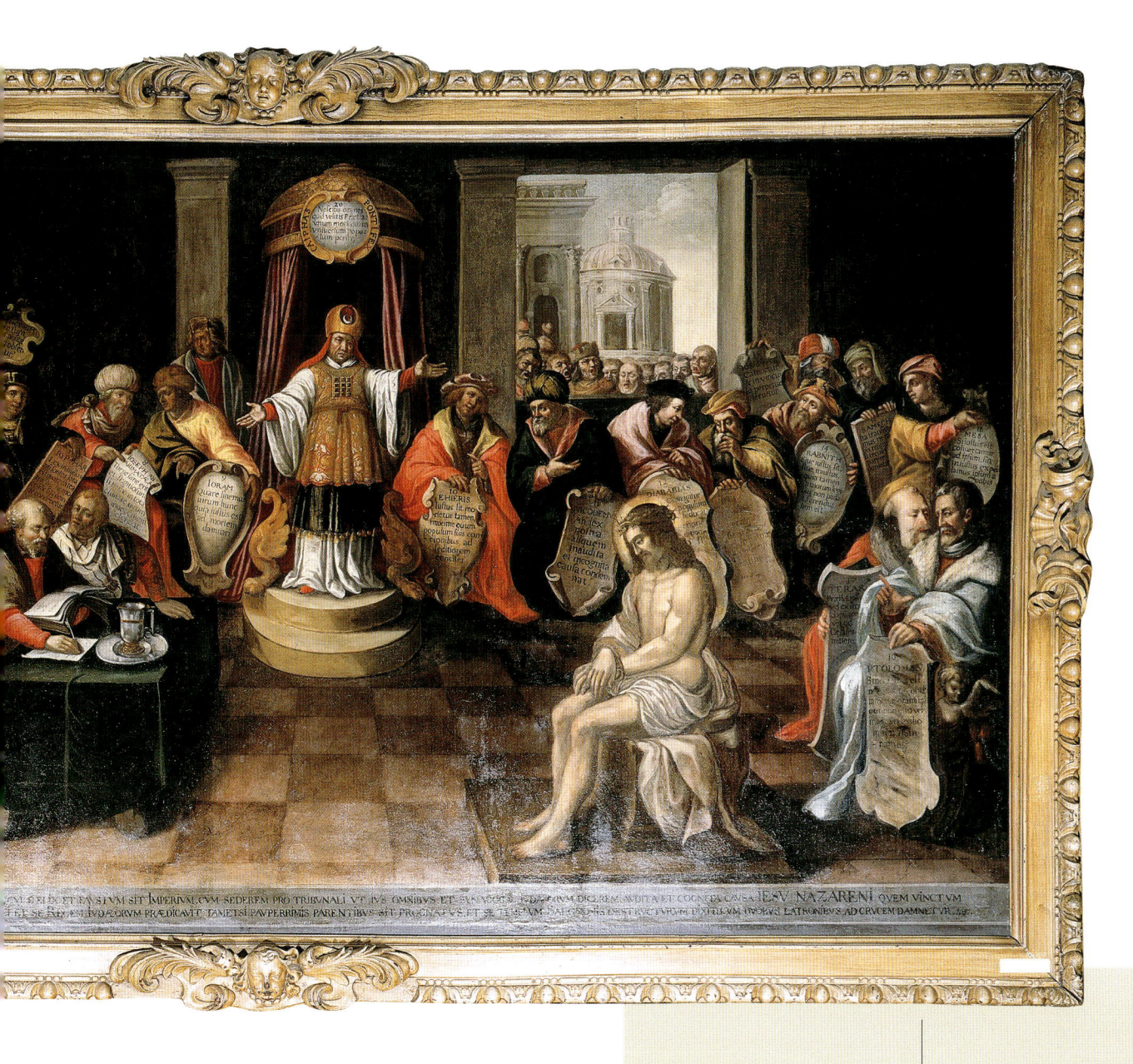

After the death of his brother Hugues, Louis Bétauld had a new ward built, dedicated to his own patron saint. He too called on the services of Isaac Moillon for the large *Death of St Louis*, signed and dated 1665.

Well known local artists from the first half of the 17th century are also represented in the painting collection. The *Annunciation* in the Salle Saint-Nicolas bears the signature of Luc Despesches just under the Virgin's work basket; and Jean Tassel is known to be the creator of *St Pelagia*, a half-length portrait whose subject, a reformed courtesan, is seen consigning her abandoned finery to an urn at the foot of a crucifix.

An odd picture in the refectory

Set into the panelling of the nuns' refectory is *Christ before Caiaphas*, a very large painting dated 1641 and showing an episode from Jesus' trial. The composition draws on Adrian Collaert's engraving after a work by Antwerp painter Martin de Vos, but its distinctive feature is the addition of the inscribed cartouches held by the numerous members of the Sanhedrin, the high court of ancient Jerusalem. The apocryphal texts give the name and opinion of each member. The carved wooden frame is decorated with cherubs' heads, palm leaves and shells.

A number of similar works are known elsewhere in France: in Côte-d'Or, Saint-Omer, Tours and Orléans.

Right: *St Martha*, second half 15th century. Facing page: *Christ of Mercy*, mid-15th century, detail. Listed as a historical monument in 1970.

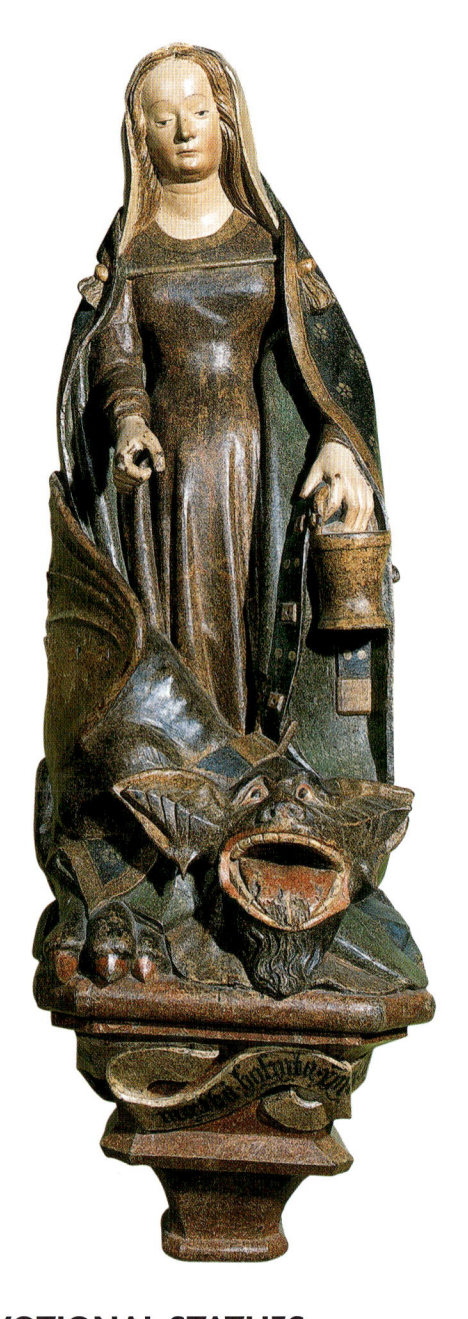

DEVOTIONAL STATUES

A poem from 1491 describes the Hôtel-Dieu as Christ's home for the poor and closes with a supplication: "Jesus Christ, compassionate redeemer, in your mercy drive back all enemy assaults on this house, that you may be served and honoured here." The prayer refers to the famous statue of Christ of Mercy in the Great Hall, surveying the room from a console above the door. Sculpted larger than life in oak, Jesus is shown seated on a piece of wood as he waits to be crucified on Golgotha, where Adam's skull is to be found. Exhausted by the Way of the Cross and his features drawn with suffering, he wears a crown of thorns and is bound hand and foot with a knotted rope; his mantle falls in smooth folds onto the rock, and a measuring device is close to hand. Unquestionably related to the images of the suffering Christ from the workshops of Brussels and Antwerp, this sculpture was probably, like the Van der Weyden polyptych, commissioned by Nicolas Rolin. A sculpture in the round from the second half of the 15th century reminds us of the Rolin family's devotion to St Martha, for whom they built chapels and commissioned works of art. One of the side altars in the Hôtel-Dieu chapel was dedicated to the saint and bore "a stone image" of her. The statue visitors now see is of painted oak, as is the scrolled console it stands on. Here the saint is shown vanquishing the tarasque, an amphibious monster, with a bucket of holy water: this is indeed part of her legend, but the gospels speak of her as serving the Lord at home and it was as the patron saint of serving women that the hospitaller nuns chose her as their protector.

St Margaret, another conqueror of dragons, was also venerated here: the 1501 inventory lists a silver reliquary containing her relics in the sacristy. However the 15th-century sculpture is from the former abbey of Sainte-Marguerite de Bouilland, and its curiously flattened appearance is explained by the fact that it was originally a double-sided relief for the choir enclosure there.

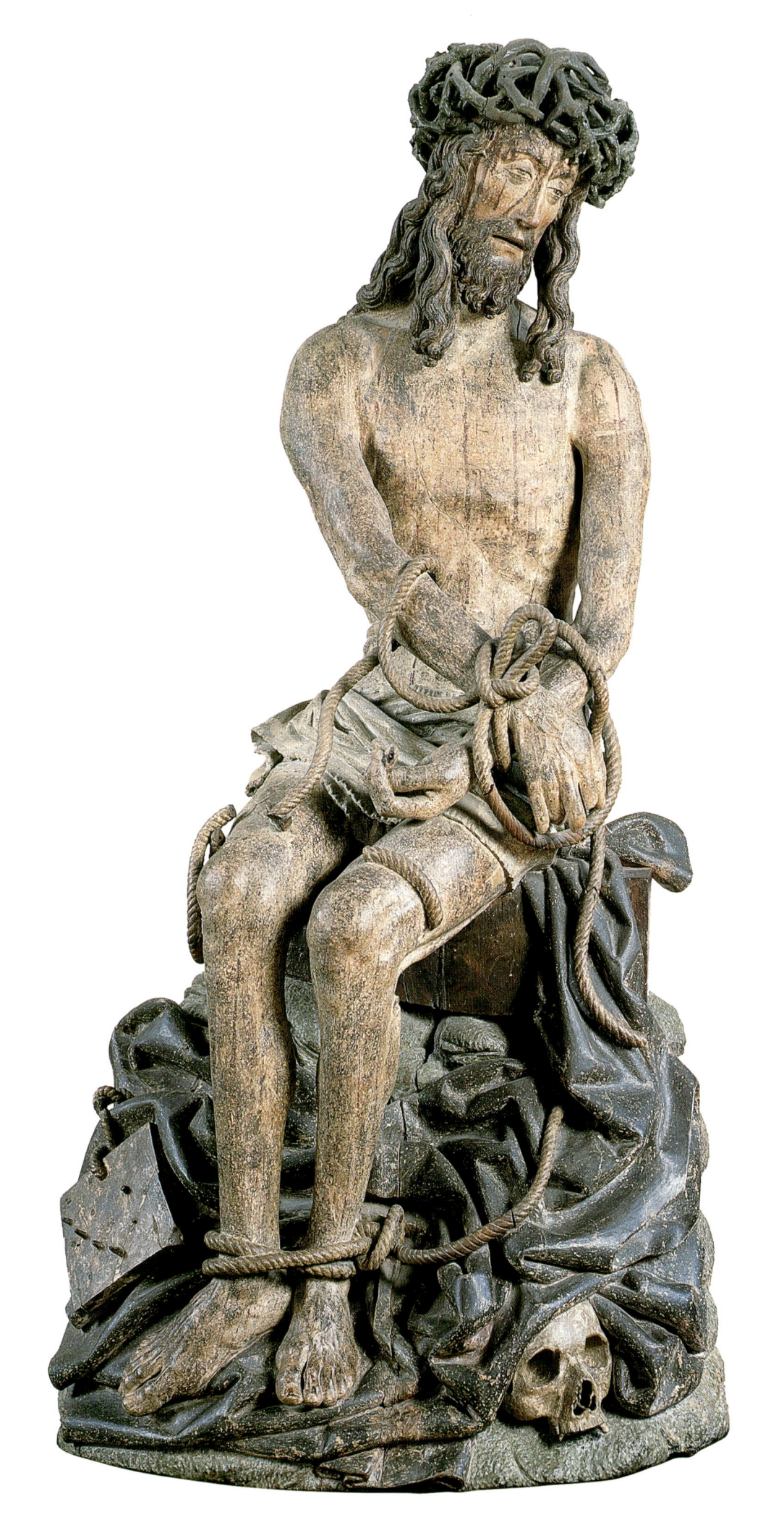

▍Right: *St John the Baptist*, early 16th century
Far right: *St Margaret*, second half 15th century.
Facing page: *St Anthony*, second half 15th century. Listed as a historical monument in 1931.

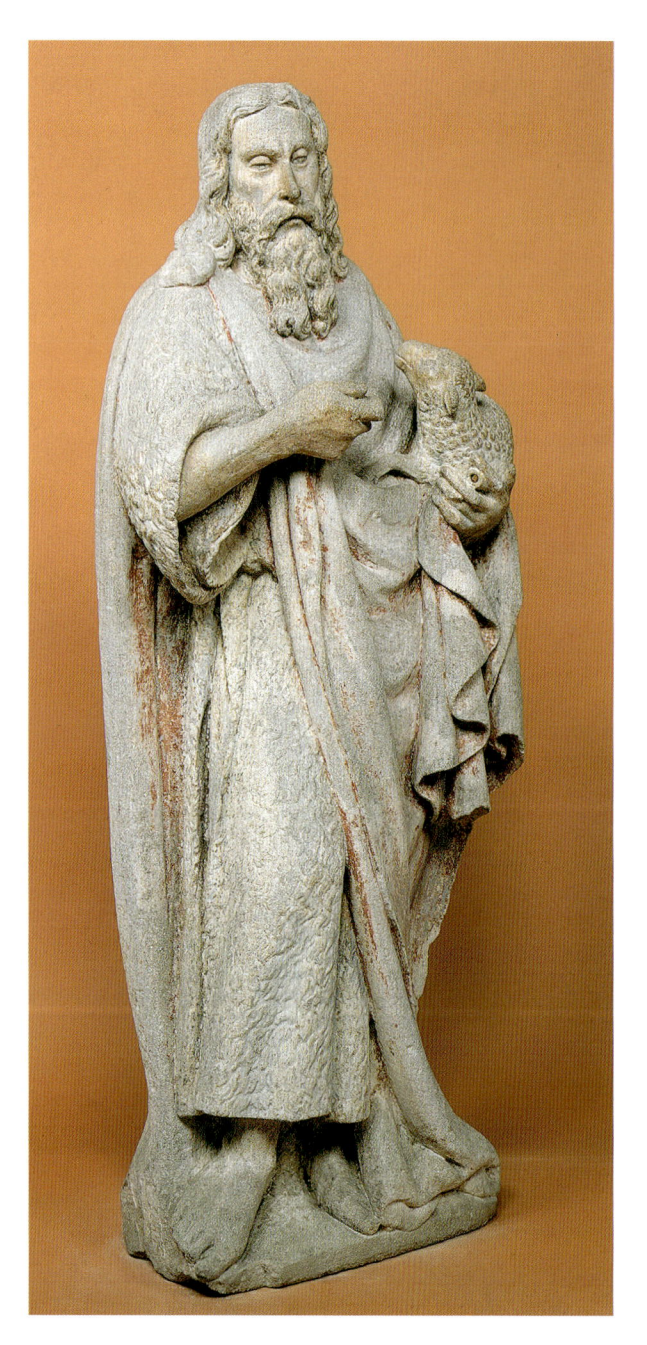

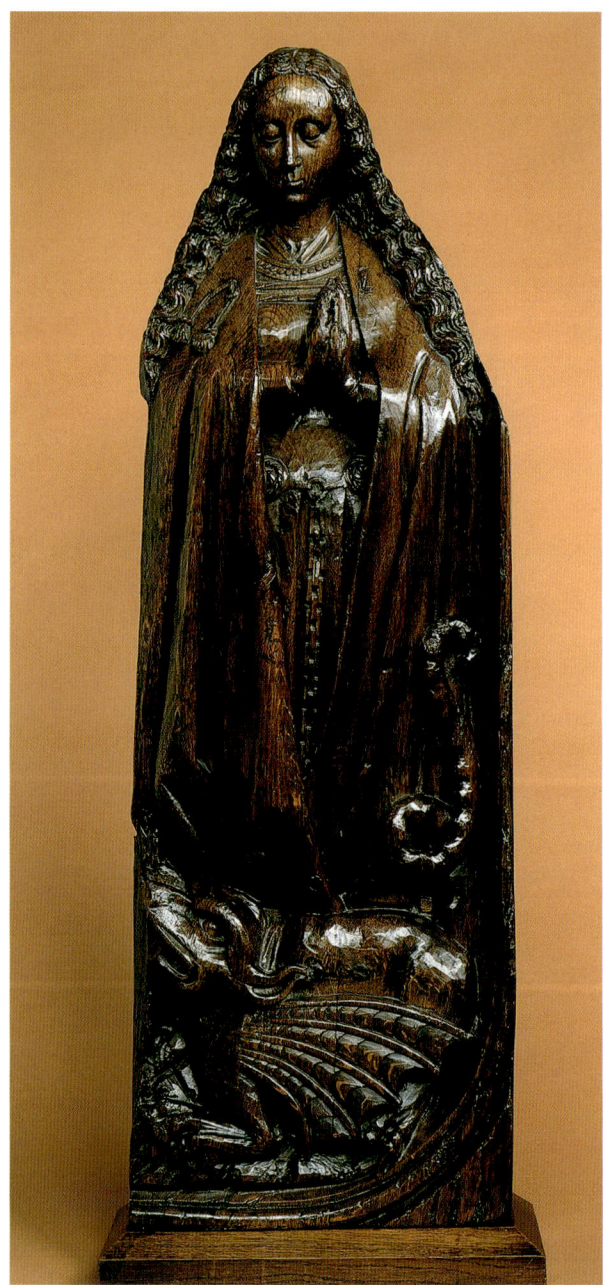

John the Baptist, the Hôtel-Dieu's second patron saint, supplanted St Anthony some ten years after the founding, in a move calculated to avoid any disputes with the Antonine order. Considered the first among all the saints, John the Baptist had been represented in the chapel since the very beginning, on both the choir enclosure and the polyptych. A reliquary bust was offered to the hospital chapel and it is known that in 1501 a "painted cloth showing the life of our lord John the Baptist" hung in the nuns' workroom. Of uncertain provenance, an early 16th-century stone statue uses the traditional image of the precursor of Christ, clad in a camel-hair tunic and pointing to the Lamb, the symbol of Christ, that he carries under his left arm.

SAINTS AND HEALERS

In the Middle Ages "antiplague" saints were especially popular because of the terror inspired by outbreaks of the disease. St Sebastian, St Anthony and Saint Roch were regarded as the most powerful intercessors in this respect and were frequently mentioned together.

In the Hôtel-Dieu's foundation charter, Chancellor Rolin specifies that he is building his hospital "in veneration and in memory of the blessed abbot Anthony and under his patronage". Made famous in the 13th century by the *Golden Legend*, this saintly healer had given his name to a host of medieval

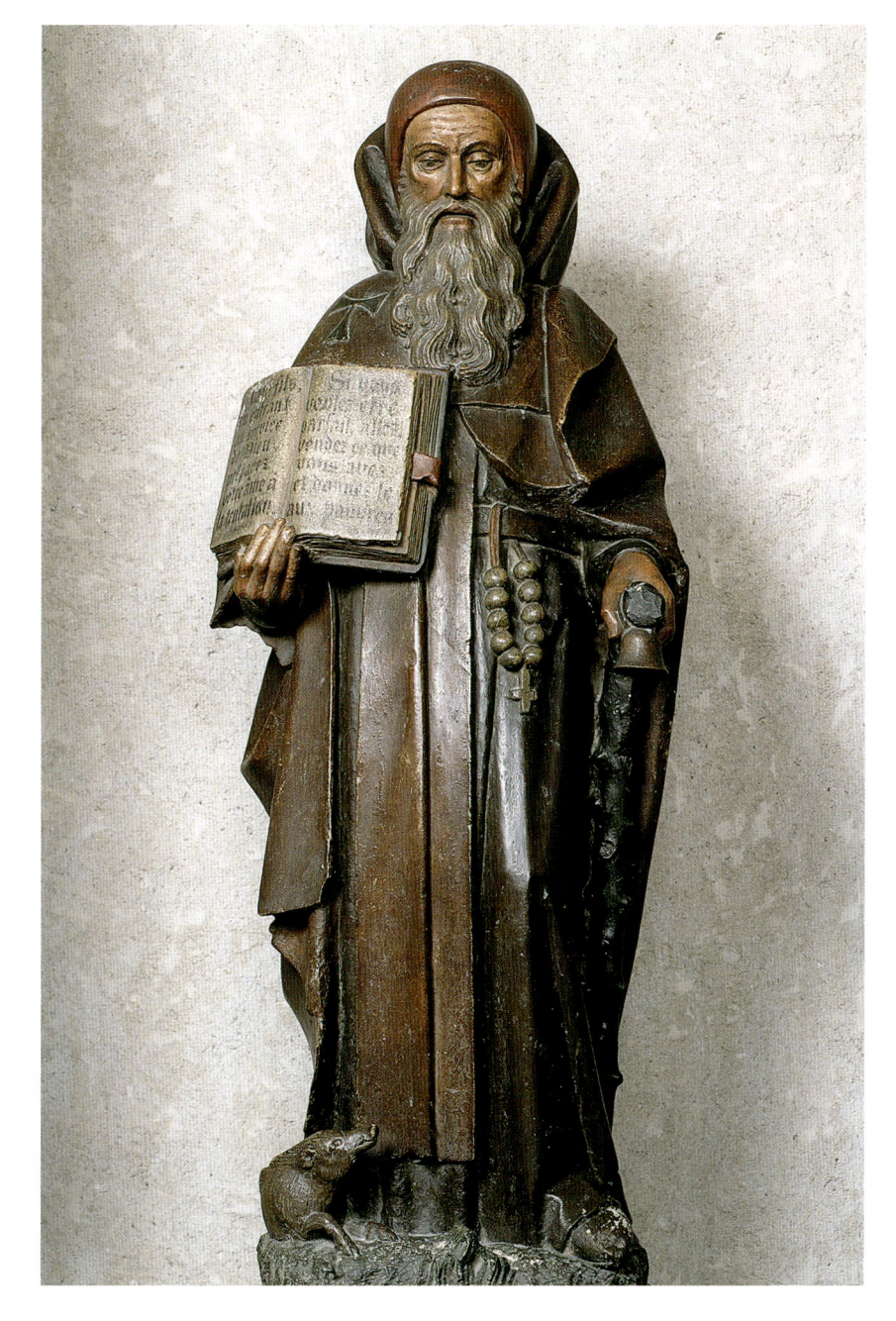

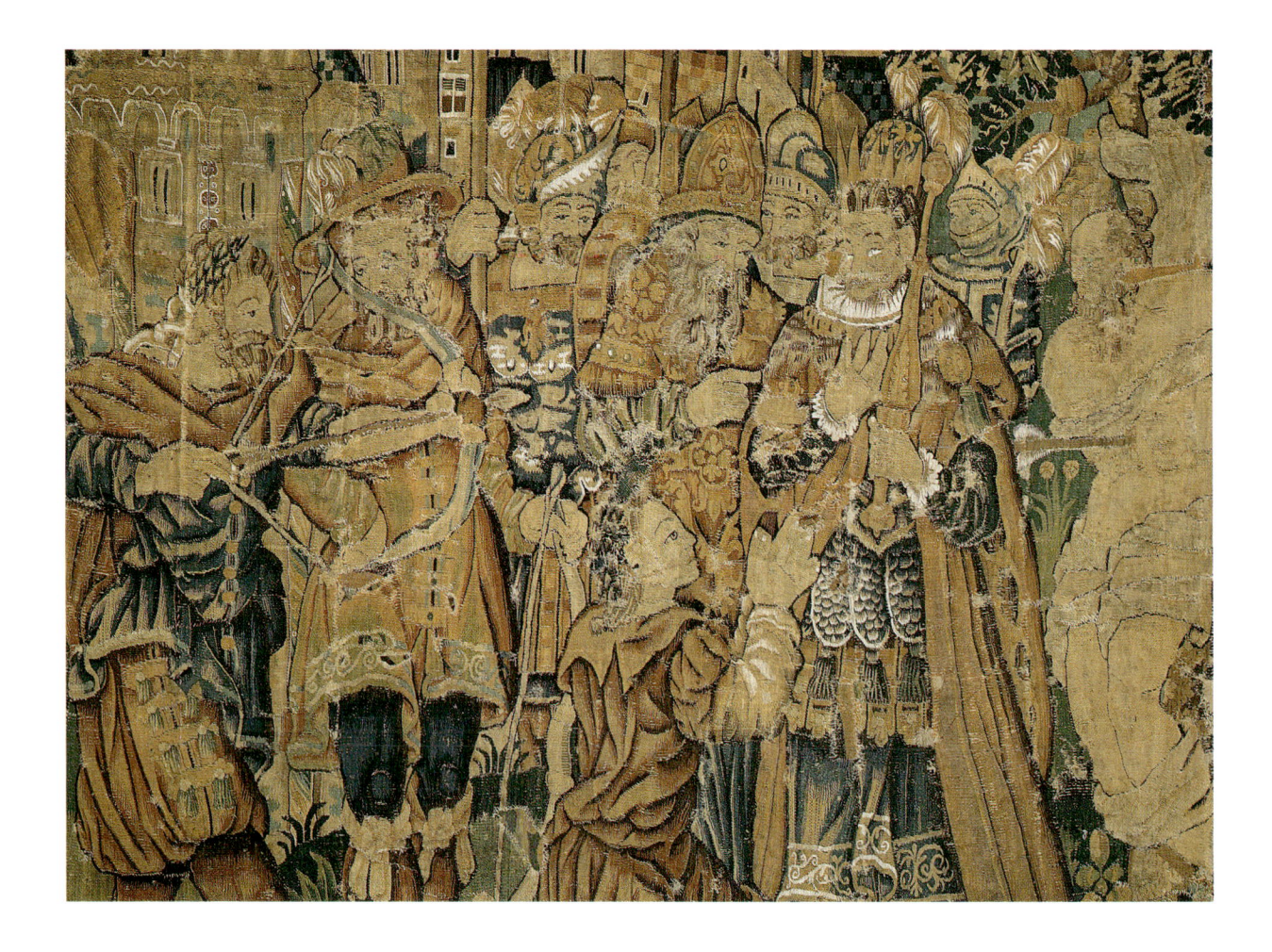

Right: *Martyrdom of St Sebastian*, tapestry, late 16th century.
Below: St Roch, wood, late 16th century.
Facing page: *Martyrdom of St Sebastian*, painting, 17th century.

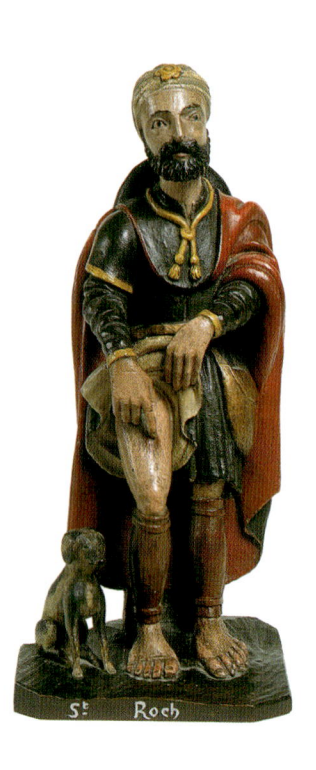

hospitals and was personally venerated by Guigone de Salins: she is shown gazing towards him in the polyptych and chose his likeness for the tapestries hung in the chapel on feast days. A statue of the saint mentioned as standing on one of the side altars may be the stone sculpture from the second half of the 15th century, in which the hermit is shown as tradition demands: in his hooded monk's habit and with a pig at his feet, he leans on a T-shaped staff with a little bell attached, surrounded by the flames of "St Anthony's fire" – the disease of ergotism, as much feared as the plague.

Like St Anthony, St Sebastian filled a dual function at the Hôtel-Dieu, as a protector against the plague and the favoured saint of the Rolin family: on the polyptych St Sebastian and the chancellor counterpoint St Anthony and Guigone de Salins. The 1501 inventory refers to a wooden statue on the altar in one of the wards: it has since disappeared, but the Hôtel-Dieu still possesses two works showing the Sebastian's martyrdom. On a fragment of late 16th-century tapestry in a curious style we see the saint pierced with arrows, but old and bearded, in accordance with the ancient tradition; by contrast a 17th-century painting offers the standard Italian version of the beardless young man.

The cult of St Roch made its appearance later, and mainly in rural areas, where he had a reputation as protecting both people and animals from epidemics. The Hôtel-Dieu has a small sculpture of him in the popular style of the late 16th century: in pilgrim's robes, the saint points to the marks of the plague on his thigh; at his side is his dog, who brought him food during his illness.

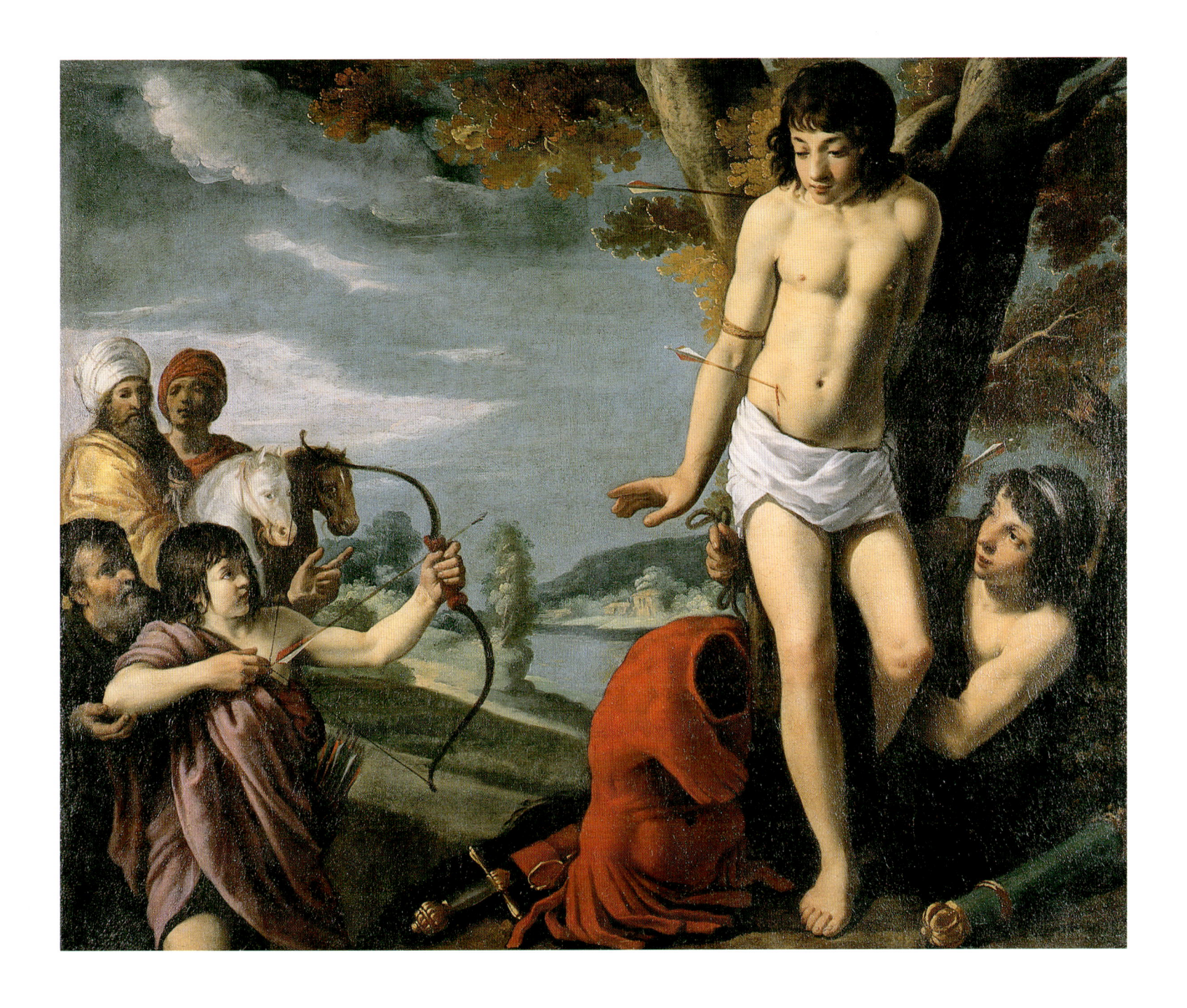

THE SACRISTY

Nicolas Rolin had provided the sacristy with sacred vessels in precious metals bearing his coat of arms, and in 1467 Guigone donated, for the chapel altar, a "most handsome gold cross" adorned with precious stones and pearls, the silver gilt base of which bore a white-enamelled gold unicorn. The cross was sold by the directors in the late 16th century.

Most of the early ritual objects have disappeared,

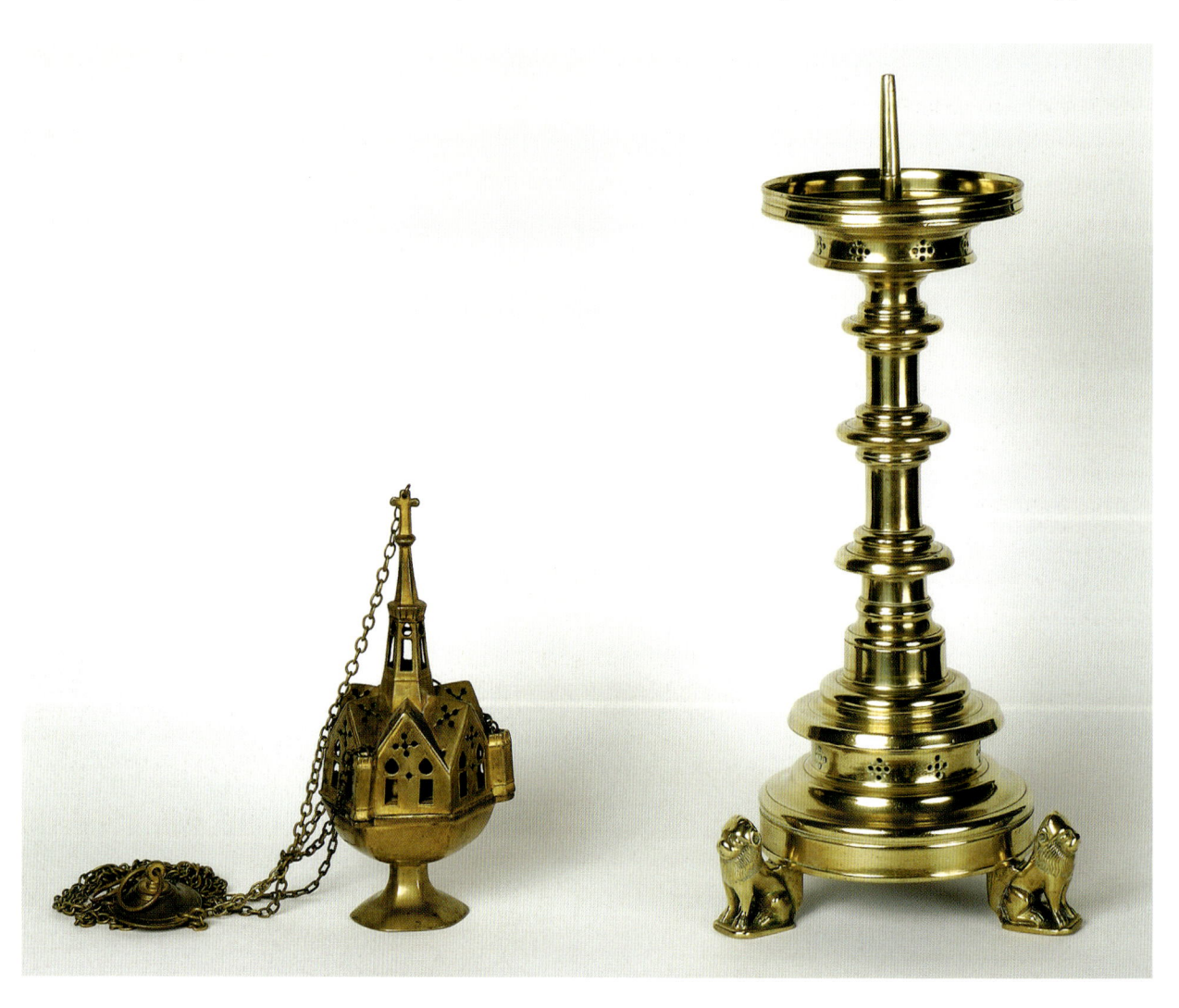

▌Right: Censer and candlestick, late 15th century.

but an altar candelabrum and a brass censer dating from the hospital's foundation have survived, doubtless because they were of baser metal. With its circular base upheld by three small lions and a stem comprising a number of turned metal rings, the candelabrum is an example of the metalwork that had become a speciality of the Burgundian Netherlands in the late 15th century. The polygonal censer has an openwork lid inspired by Gothic steeples and may be one of the four brass censers mentioned in the inventory of 1501.

The Antoine de Salins bell

Doubtless coeval with the founding of the hospital, a bell some forty centimetres high bears in Gothic lettering the inscriptions SANCTI SPIRITUS SIT NOBIS GRATIA AMEN and A DE SALINS together with the latter's coat of arms. Dean of the chapter of the collegiate church of Notre-Dame de Beaune and a member of Guigone's family, Antoine de Salins was probably one of the Hôtel-Dieu's benefactors. Did this clock, now removed from its original setting, ring out from the belltower? Or did it sound the call to meals at the entrance to the Great Hall, as the 1501 inventory indicates?

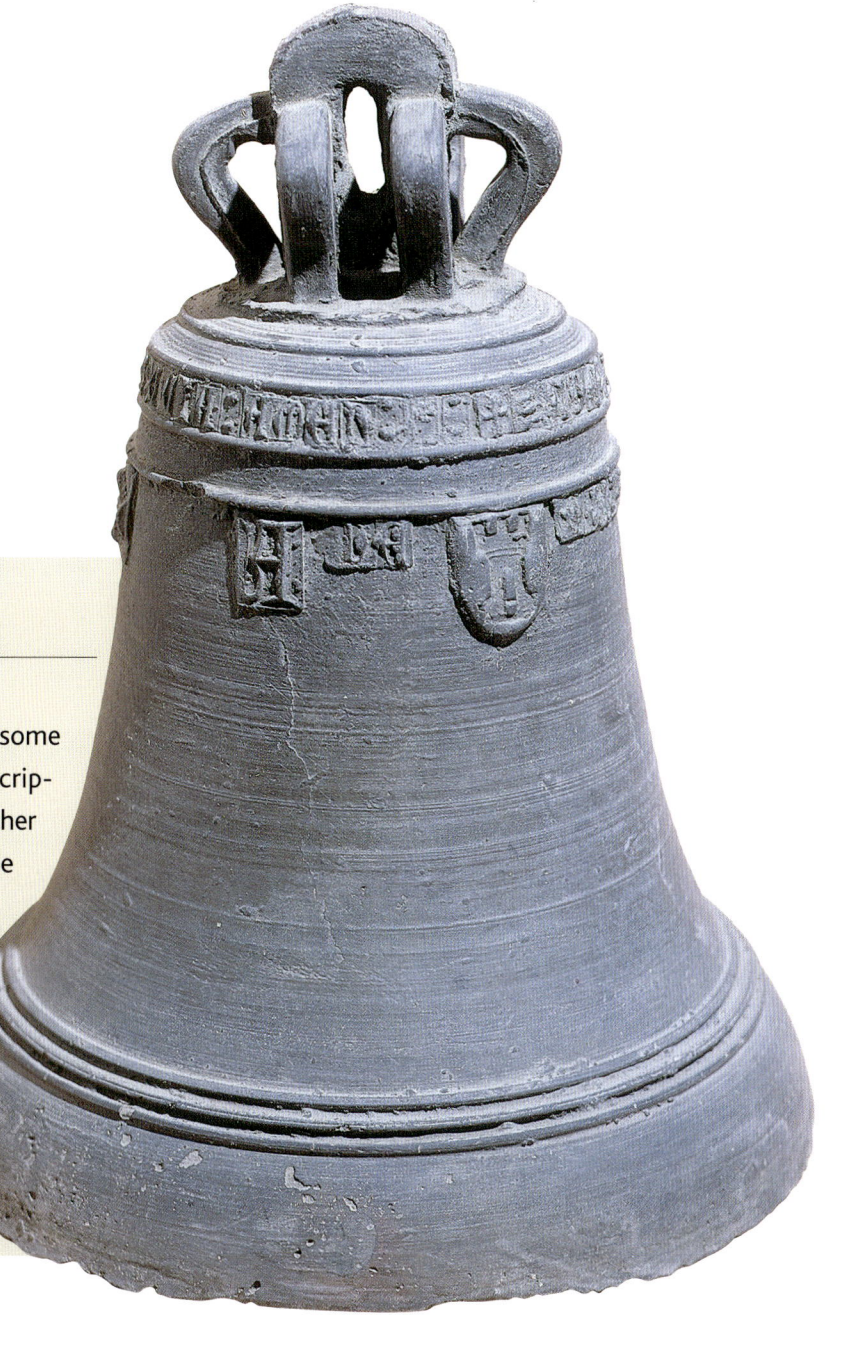

Women and men at the service of the sick

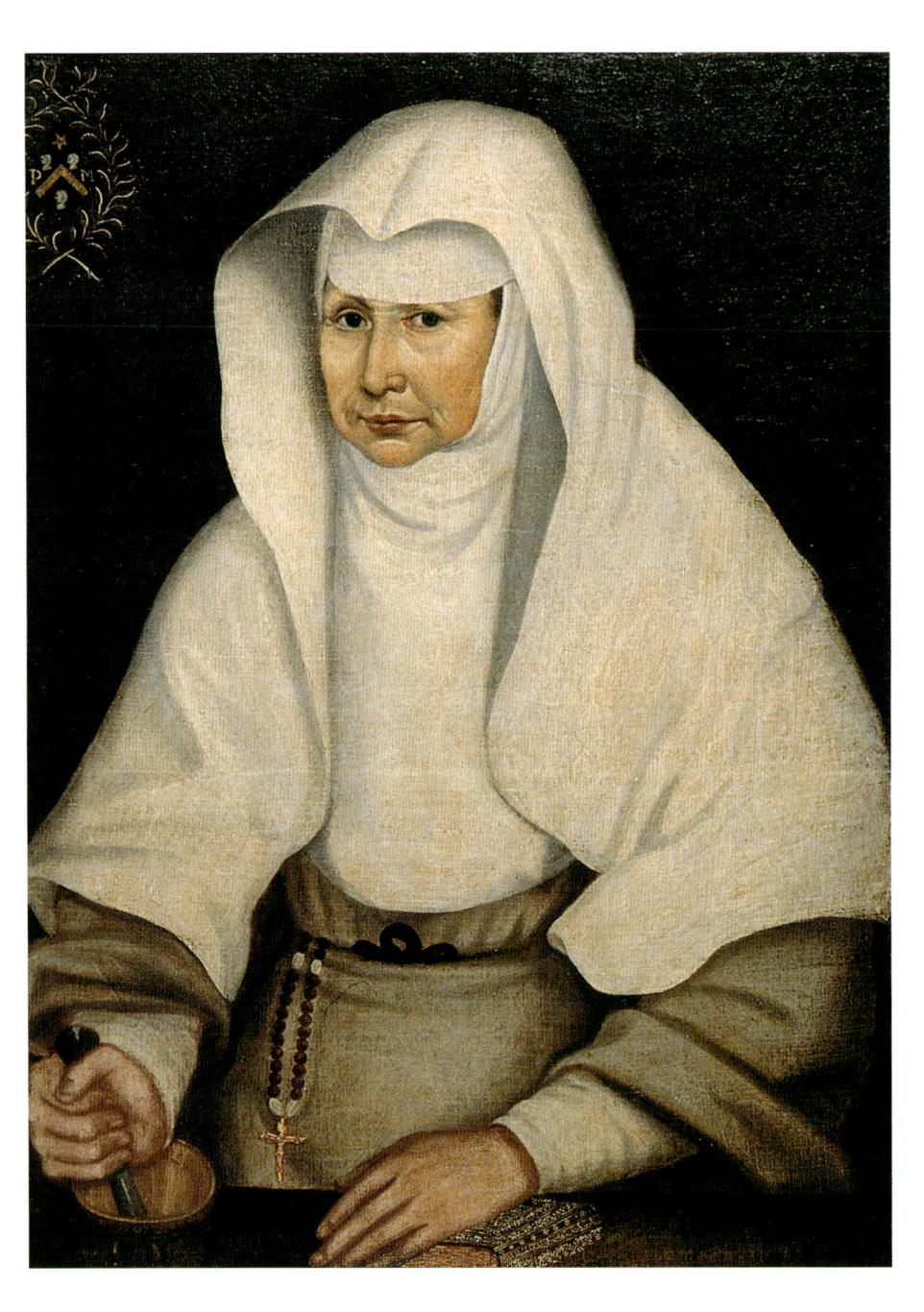

THE HOSPITALLER NUNS

For the care of the patients, Nicolas Rolin had called on six nuns from the hospital at Valenciennes. They brought their order's rule with them, but the chancellor, finding it inappropriate, drew up another for which he gained papal approval in 1459. The vows were simple: poverty, chastity and obedience "for as long as they resided in the House". The rule required that "they be diligent in their duty towards the poor in all their needs, both bodily and spiritual" and that they care for them "with pious compassion, true zeal and a countenance as joyous as possible". After the death of Guigone de Salins the nuns elected their own directress, until then appointed by the secular head of the hospital. The community hived off forty-six others in France and five in Switzerland. The rule excluded perpetual vows and remained in force until 1939; and until the mid-20th century the sisters retained their quaint medieval costume of a robe with a train and the high conical hennin of white cloth. Some of them continue to work today in the hospital or with the aged.

Portraits of nuns have come down to us as testimony to the commitment of these "devout women" who gave their lives to the care of the sick. Although the paintings cover the period from the 17th to the 20th century, the composition remains constant: a half-length portrait, usually in three-quarter view. The oldest, dating from 1624, is of sister Monet, who died

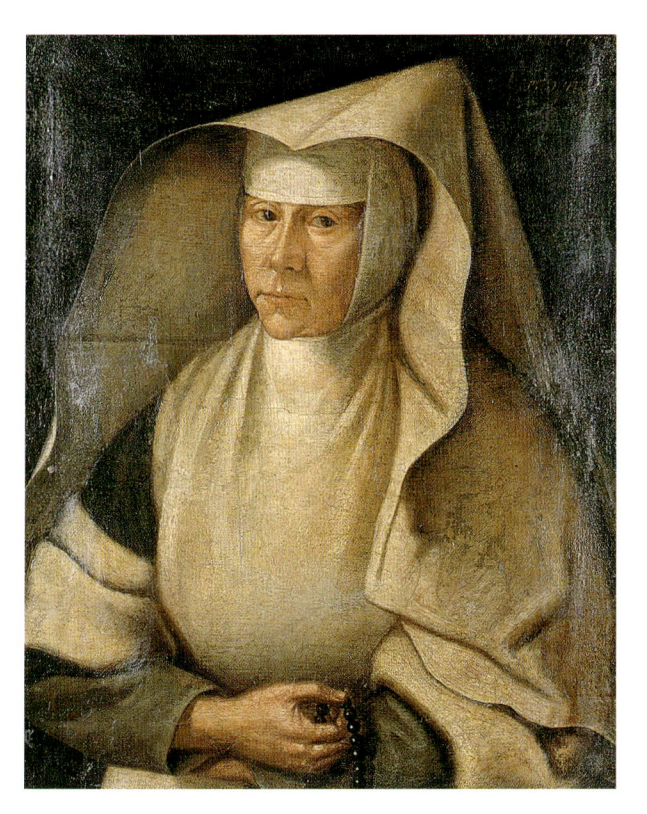

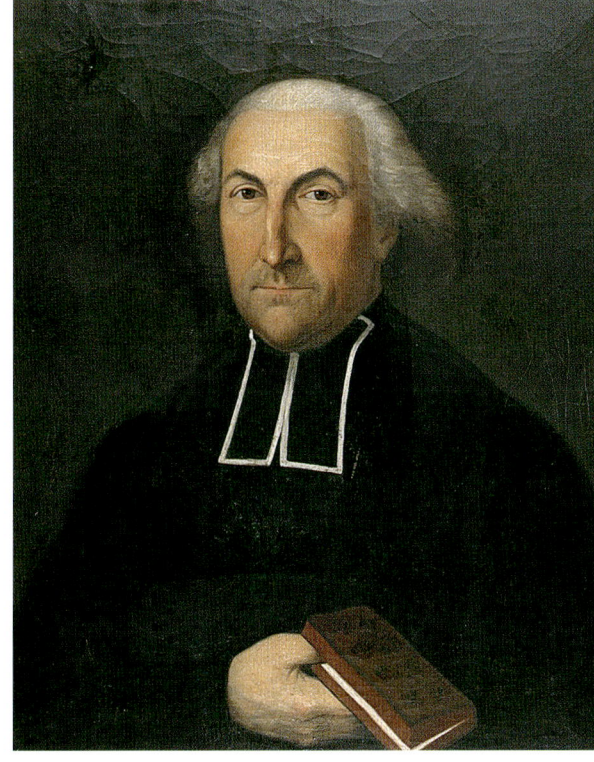

Facing page: Portrait of Sister Monet, 1624.
Far Left: Portrait of Sister Lemoyne, 1624.
Left: Portrait of Abbé Forien, early 19th century.

of plague four years later: she is shown with a mortar, the symbol of her role as apothecary. Sister Marguerite Lemoyne, portrayed in 1677 at the age of fifty, is saying her rosary. Imprisoned during the Revolution, sister Suzanne Brunet appears in a portrait painted after her return to the community.

While Chancellor Rolin took great care to provide the hospital with competent staff, he retained for himself and his heirs the right to make and revoke appointments. He had a very clear idea of the contribution each member of staff should make to the efficient running of his establishment: "I have also ordered that mass be said every day and in perpetuity, in the presence of the poor, and that the sacraments of the Church be administered to them by capable chaplains...A master or rector and a treasurer for the hospital, with nuns to take care of the poor...A directress in charge of the aforementioned nuns and a confessor to hear their confession."

The spiritual life of the nuns was entrusted to "fathers" serving as superior and confessor. The celebration of religious rites having been banned under

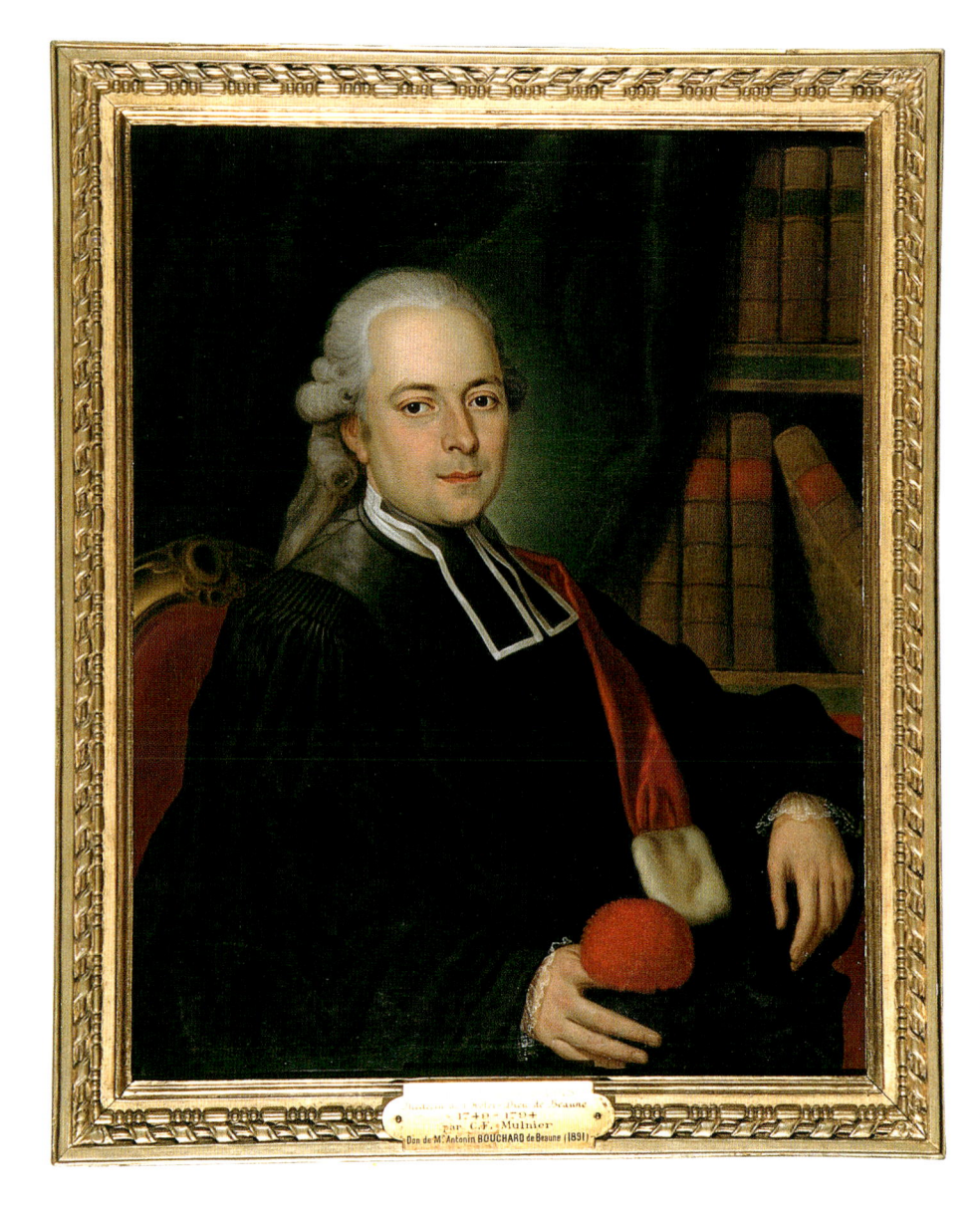

Several dynasties of doctors came and went, among them the Morelots and the Bourgeois in the 18th century and the Leflaives in the 19th. Some of them we know via their portraits, the most remarkable of which is that of Jean-Baptiste Bourgeois by Charles-Félix Mulnier, official painter to Stanislas Leszczyński, king of Poland. Bourgeois, who continued to practise until 1794, is shown wearing the garb of his profession, with bands, red scarf and red-pompommed hat.

■ Above: Portrait of Dr Bourgeois by Charles-Félix Mulnier, 18th century.
Right: Portrait of Jean de Massol, dated 1646.

the Revolution, Abbé Forien, appointed to this post in 1790, officially returned to his functions at the Hôtel-Dieu in 1802.

THE DOCTORS

No provision had been made in the charter for the post of doctor. For everyday care the nuns prepared the medicines or called on Beaune's barber-surgeons and doctors. Later the hospital appointed its own physicians.

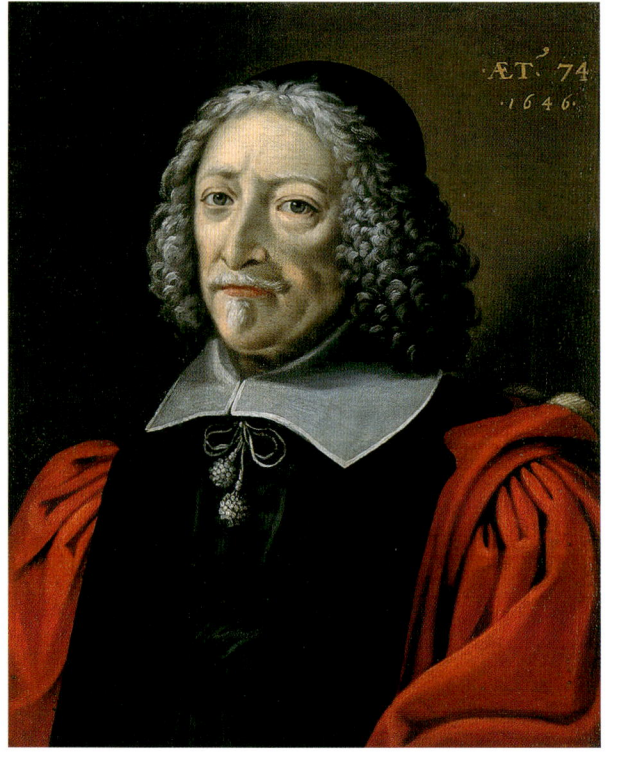

THE BENEFACTORS

The hospital was aided by the generosity of numerous benefactors, civil servants and members of Parliament, whose gifts allowed for the construction of new buildings, the furnishing and decoration of the wards and the creation of new beds. In 1669 Jean de Massol, a member of the Parliament of Burgundy, bequeathed all his property to the poor of the hospital: his portrait dating from 1646 and that of his small daughter have been given a place of honour in the Chambre du Roi.

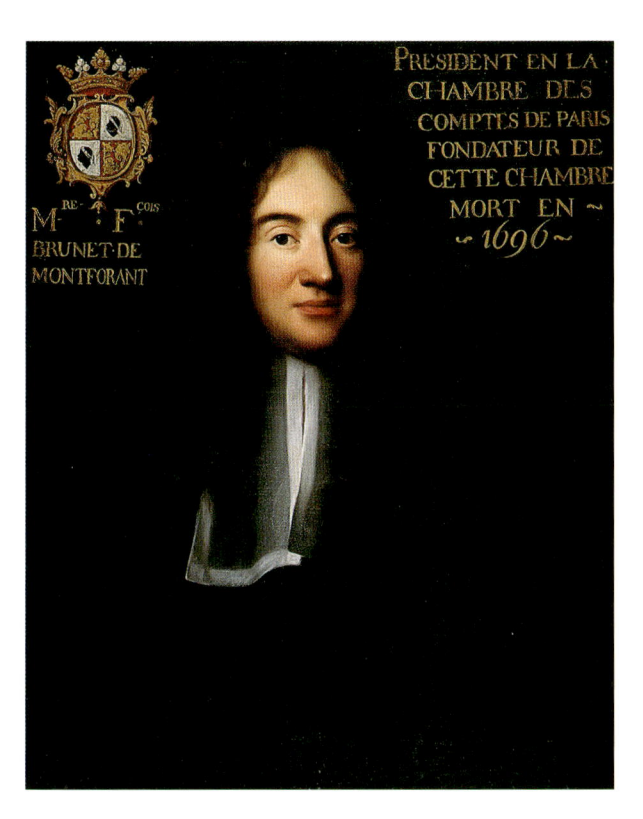

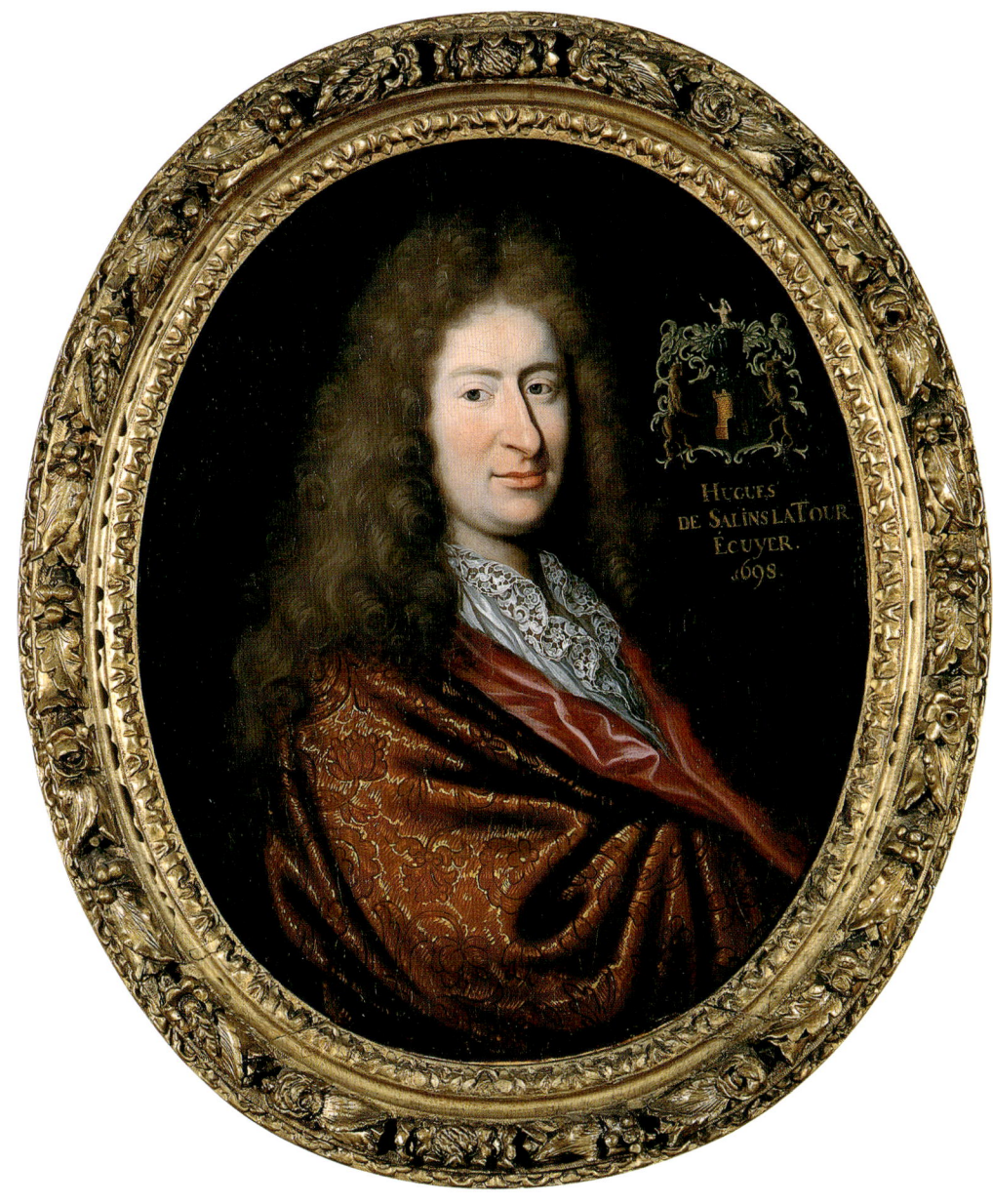

In the same room are ceremonial portraits of François Brunet de Montforand and Hugues de Salins La Tour, with their coats of arms. The former, a high-ranking financial official in Paris, endowed three beds in the Salle Sainte-Anne; when he died his heart was buried there and the ward became the Salle Saint-François. A descendent of the Hôtel-Dieu's founders, Hugues de Salins La Tour is presented in an oval frame carved with plant motifs.

▌Left: Portrait of Brunet de Montforand, who died in 1690.
Above: Portrait of Hugues de Salins La Tour, dated 1698.

Functional furnishings

Nicolas Rolin drew up the hospital's statutes and rules in August 1459, insisting that the overseer make an annual check of the condition of all furnishings. The earliest inventories have never been found. The oldest of those now in the Hôtel-Dieu archives– it bears the title *Inventory of the property, furniture and other things presently belonging to the great hospital of Beaune* – dates from 1501 and was regularly updated over the years 1507-21. The furniture and other objects in each room are methodically described and some of them can be recognised among the pieces making up today's Hospices de Beaune collection. Religious material was listed first, followed by the domestic furnishings: beds and their accessories, seats and tables, and such storage furniture as chests, linen cupboards and sideboards.

The inventory makes it clear that each ward had its own furniture and utensils and there was no mixing or exchange. The nuns carried on this tradition and until the middle of the 20th century all furniture and other items were stamped with the mark of the room they belonged to (see box, p. 98).

BEDS FOR THE POOR

For the Great Hall of the Poor the inventory makes mention of thirty-one beds, each comprising a bedstead topped with an open canopy whose uprights were carved with two little statues. The beds, set on a kind of wooden platform, could be closed off with two white curtains hung from the canopy. There were benches too, serving as seats, shelves and perhaps also as a step.

As was frequently the case in medieval hospitals, the beds were placed perpendicular to the side walls of the ward, beside niches in the masonry.

Successive changes, notably the major restoration carried out by Maurice Ouradou in 1874-78, left little trace of this original arrangement: the chapel enclosure was brought further forward into the Great Hall, new beds were made running parallel to the side walls and benches were installed in the *ruelle* between the beds and the wall.

The other wards usually contained wooden bedsteads, together with extra bunks and camp beds. In some cases they were topped with a wood and fabric canopy hung from four iron hooks set in the ceiling, while their drapes or curtains ran on iron rails concealed behind strips of material. The colours of the fittings varied according to the wards: red for the ground floor ward, the Chambre-Dieu and the Chambre de la Croix; violet in the patients' infirmary and the Salle Sainte-Marthe, green in the Salle Saint-Jean and white in the nuns' infirmary. The Salle Notre-Dame had chequered blankets and others decorated with oak leaves, the oak being Chancellor Rolin's emblematic plant.

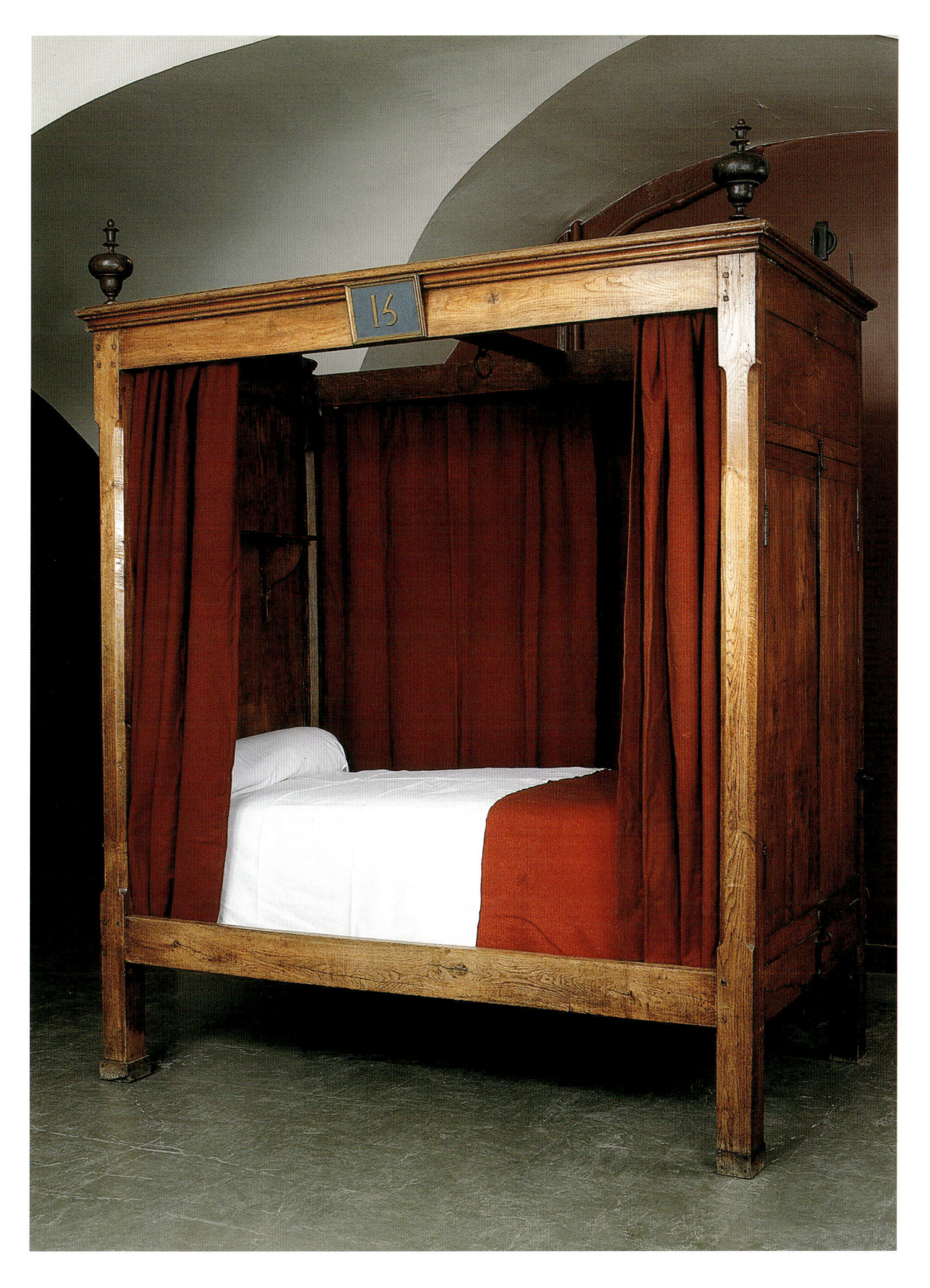

Bed, 17th century.

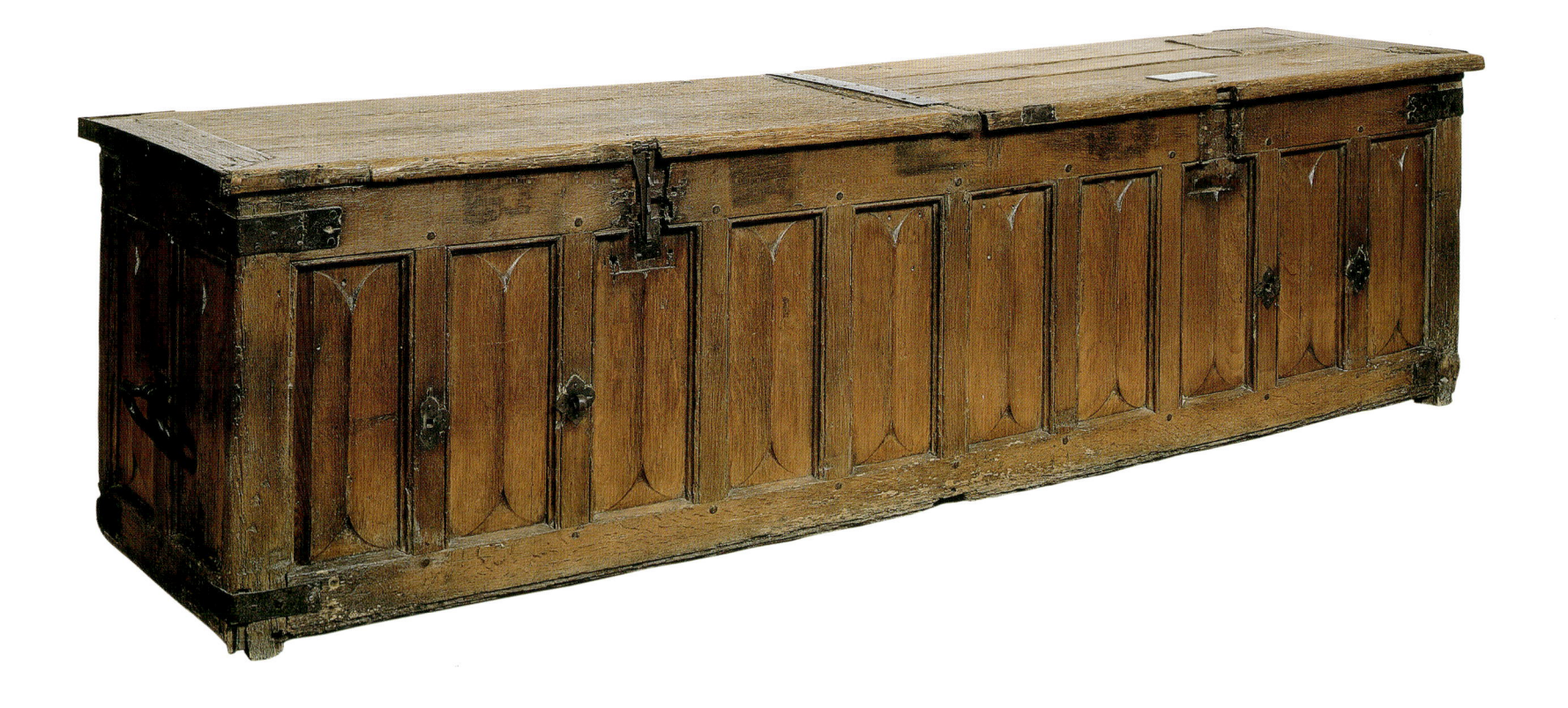

■ Above: Linen chest with two compartments, mid-15th century.
Facing page: Chest decorated with blind tracery, mid-15th century.
Following pages:
Page 96: Cupboard with diamond fret pattern, late 17th or early 18th century. Linen cupboard with curved Rococo panels, late 18th century.
Page 97: Upper left: Grain or flour chest, second half 15th century.
Upper right: Ironbound chest, mid-15th century.
Bottom: Four-doored linen cupboard, first half 18th century.

The rooms with two to four beds were all furnished in the same way: a two-part sideboard – a lower shelf for the crockery and an upper part with a single drawer – with one or two doors; in front of the fire, a turning bench whose movable back meant one could sit facing the fire but have one's back to it when eating; and at least one table with six or eight rectangular stools. The linen was kept in ordinary chests, in chest-steps placed by the beds, and in other chests that also served as benches.

FROM CHESTS TO CUPBOARDS

The chest was the means of storage par excellence from the Middle Ages to the mid-18th century, when it was systematically replaced by the cupboard. Few hospitals have kept their chests, but the Hospices de Beaune still have a hundred or so. Among the thirty-five dating from the 15th century are seven two-compartment models, their panels lined with parchment, that held linen in various wards. The observer notices a clear kinship between the furniture and the door frames in the original buildings, indicating that they were part of an overall aesthetic agenda and were made by the same tradesmen.

The chests sculpted with blind tracery are mentioned in the inventories for the storage of precious objects and books.

A pair of ironbound chests with hasp locks was most probably ordered as maximum security storage for valuable items. Handles on each side meant they could be moved about as necessary.

Other, more simple chests – called *arches* in French – were used for storing foodstuffs. Practical and not designed to be moved about, they had massive

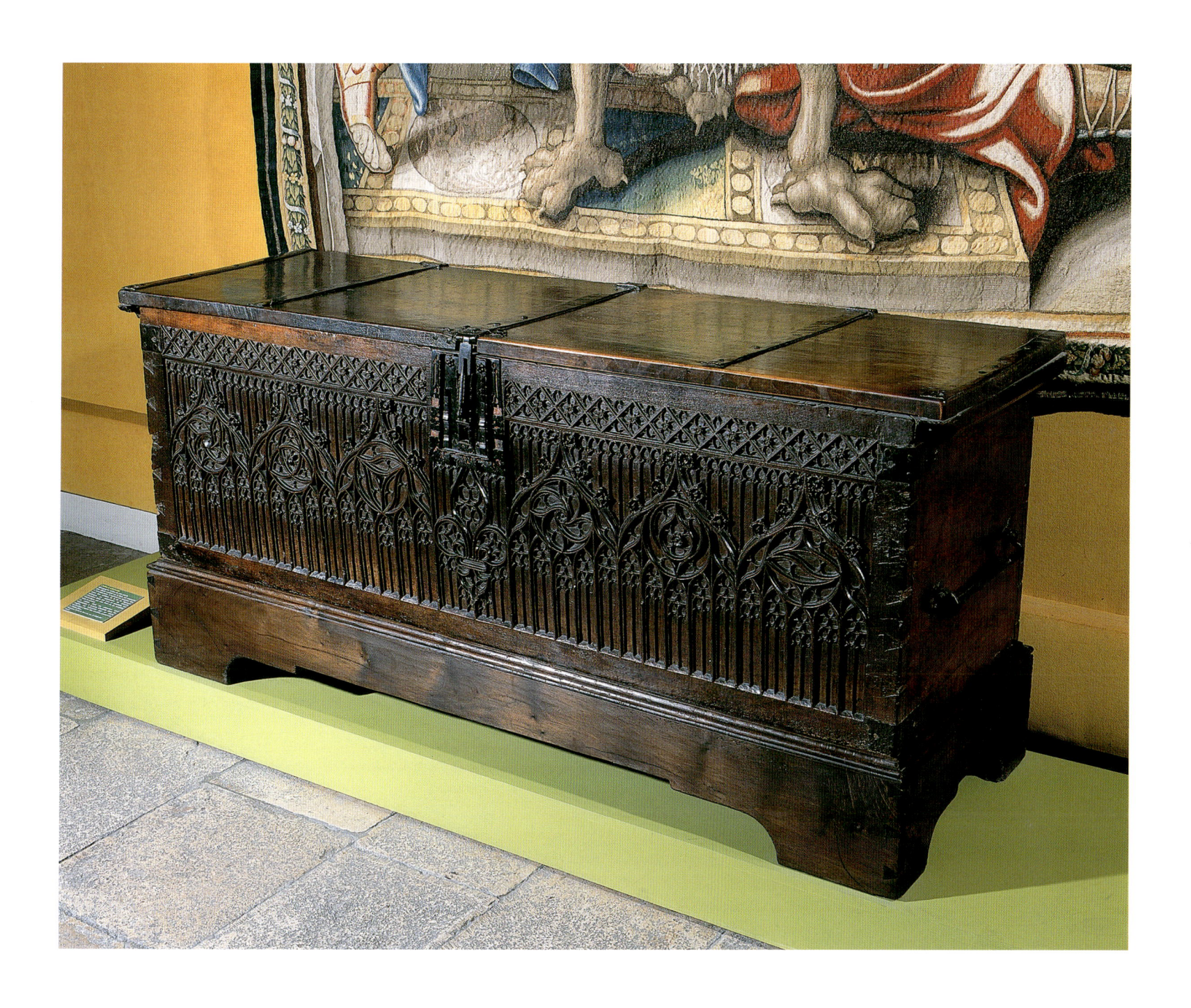

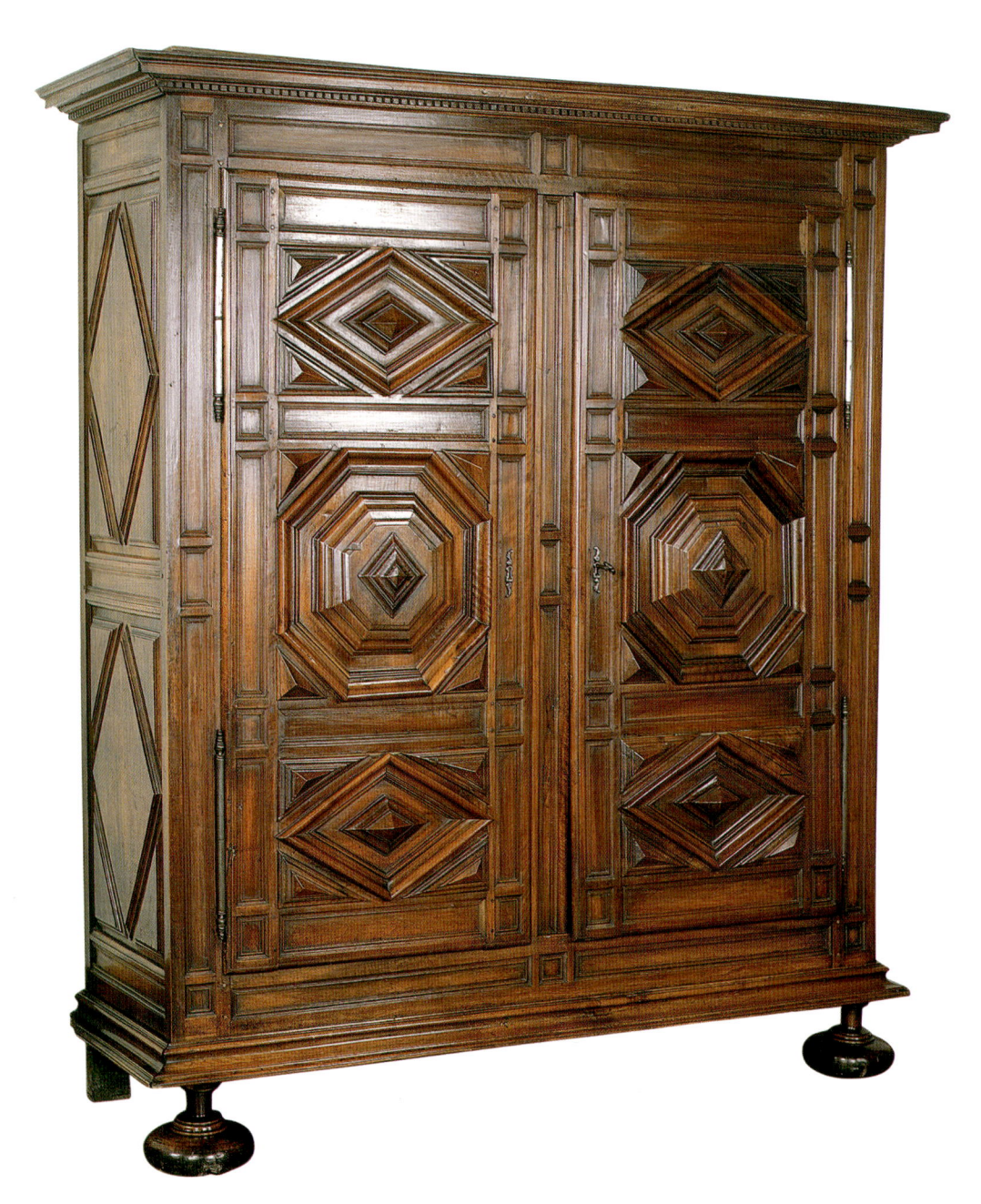

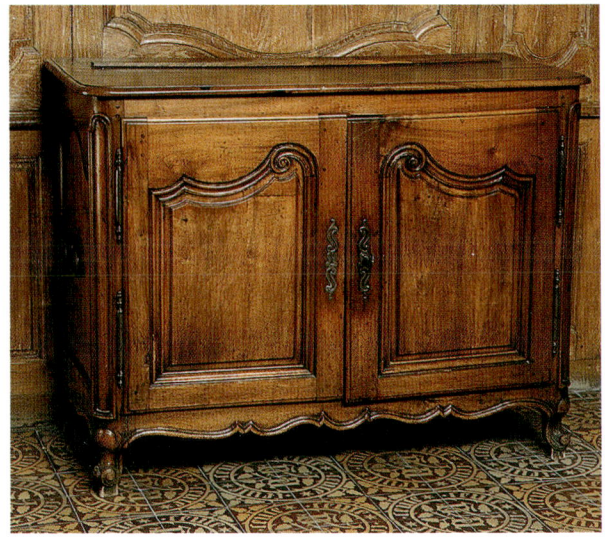

rectangular legs supporting a box each of whose panels was made of a single plank. Of variable quality, the oak used had been sawn then planed. On the front of one of them Guigone de Salins' coat of arms – the tower and three keys – has been burnt in. The two chests that originally flanked the entrance to the Great Hall were replaced in the early 18th century by two low, four-door walnut cupboards serving exactly the same purpose. The commonest storage pieces in the 18th century were little cupboards with curved Rococo panels, which the nuns continued to refer to as "chests".

As the hospital furnishings were counted in with the domestic equipment, it is not easy to know which came from donations, which from bequests and

97

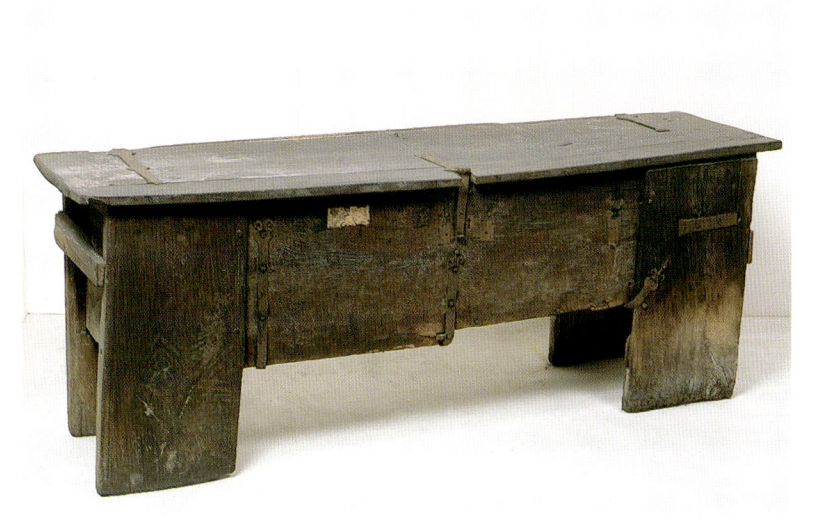

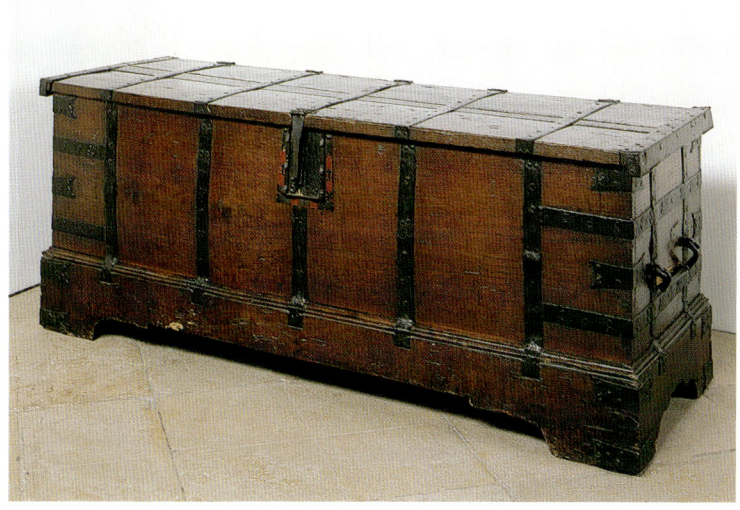

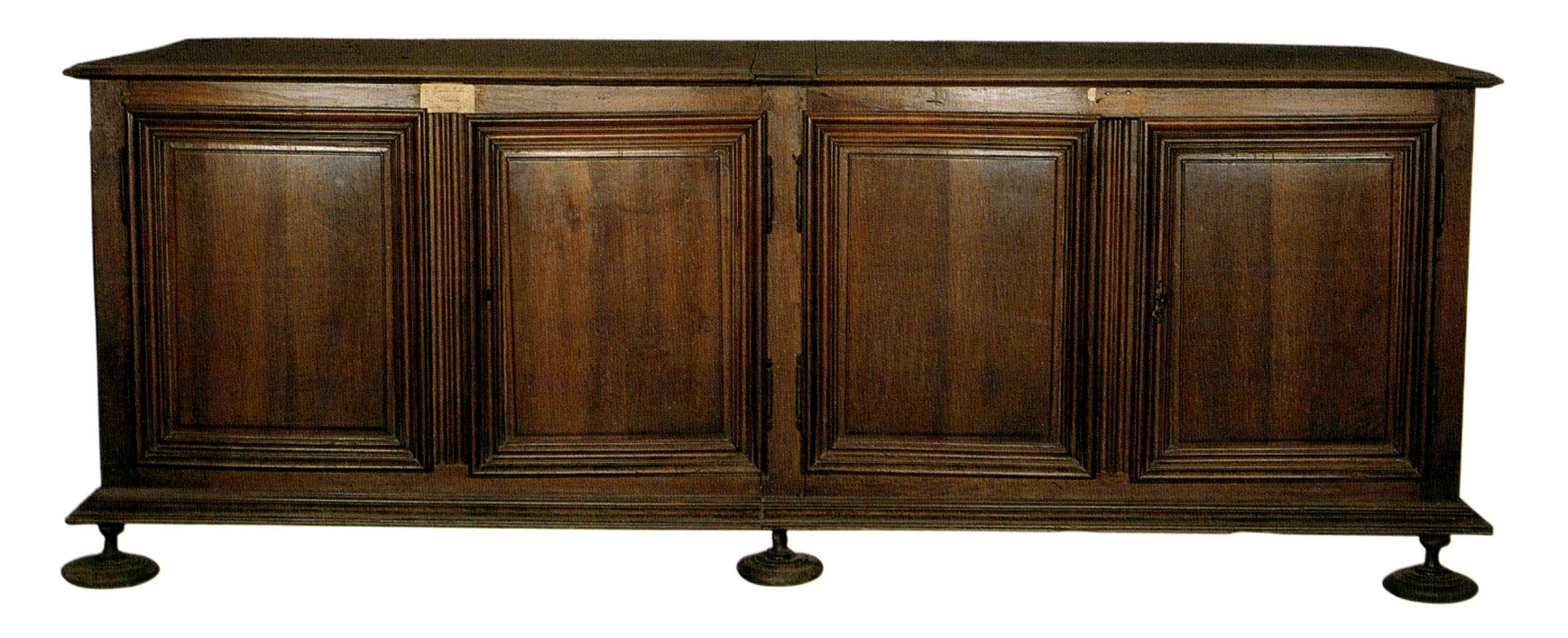

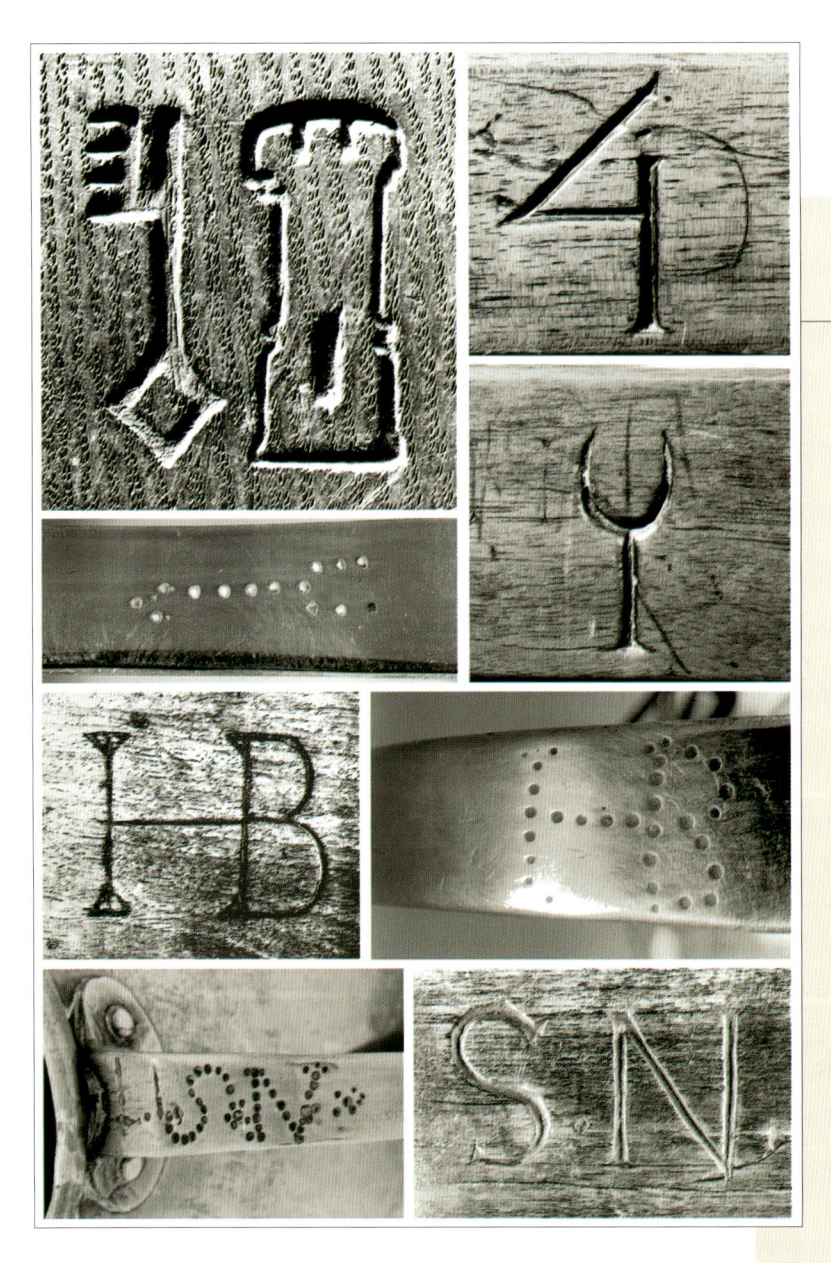

Marking the furniture

The hospital's solution to the problem of monitoring its furniture and domestic equipment was a system of marking that meant each piece of furniture and each everyday item had its own place. Initials or symbols indicating the room the piece belonged to were cut into the upper rung of the chairbacks or stamped on the handles of ladles and jugs: the figure 4 for the Great Hall, the initials H.B. (Hugues Bétauld) for the Salle Saint-Hugues, S.N. for the Salle Saint-Nicolas, S.F. for the Salle Saint-François and a two-pronged fork for the kitchen. Most of the surviving markings are no earlier than the 17th or 18th centuries, but the system seems to go back to the founding of the hospital: the 1501 inventory mentions, in the Great Hall, tablecloths "all bearing the mark of the aforementioned room".

Hôtel-Dieu still has a fine 17th-century example. The tables on which the patients' meals were served were usually smaller and made according to a single model. The most frequent survivor among the medical furnishings is the commode, which took the form of a stool, chair or armchair. In each case a lid covered a seat with a circular opening above a metal or ceramic bucket. The Hospices de Beaune have a fine collection dating from the 17th to the 20th century.

The furnishings from the dispensary and the pharmacy are usually in two sections: the lower one, or drug cabinet, contained the most commonly used ingredients, while the upper – called the powder cabinet, or shelf – housed the ceramic (and later, glass) pots. There were also specific pieces of furniture for the preparation of medicine in the laboratory or "kitchen" off the pharmacy. Two cupboards dated 1585 and 1674 can be identified as having served for the storage of medicines: each has numerous sliding shelves behind two folding doors hinged down the middle.

In the late 15th and early 16th centuries the patients were brought to the hospital on a litter mentioned in the 1501 inventory. A mid-18th-century sedan chair serving the same purpose can still be seen in the Hôtel-Dieu, whose coat of arms is painted on the back.

Inside the hospital, the means of transport were stretchers, wheeled beds or wheelchairs. Chair-stretchers were used for going up and down stairs.

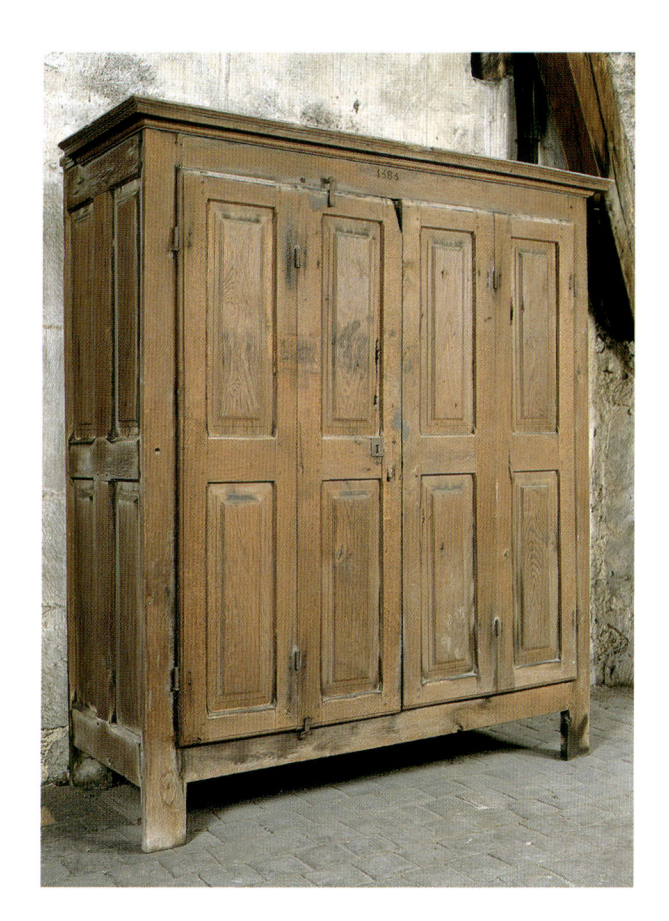

which from the nuns' families. Some of the numerous cupboards are decorated with a sophisticated diamond fret pattern.

CARE AND NOURISHMENT

In the hospitals of the time the kitchens needed narrow tables up to five metres long, of which the

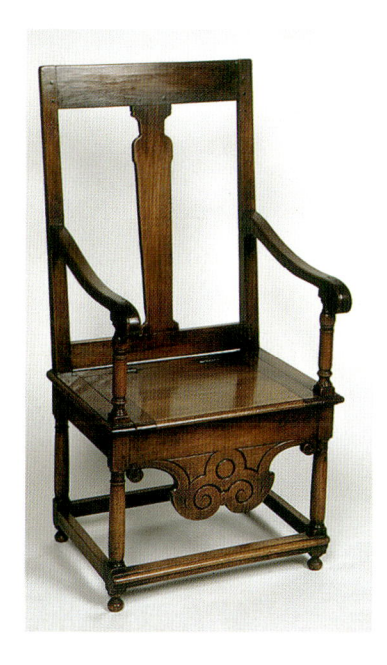

■ Left: Medicine cupboard, dated 1585.
Above: Commode, second half 17th century.

Right: Sedan chair, mid-18th century.
Far right: A *guérite*, late 17th or early 18th century.
Facing page: Dove tapestry, between 1443 and 1462. Listed as a historical monument in 1943.

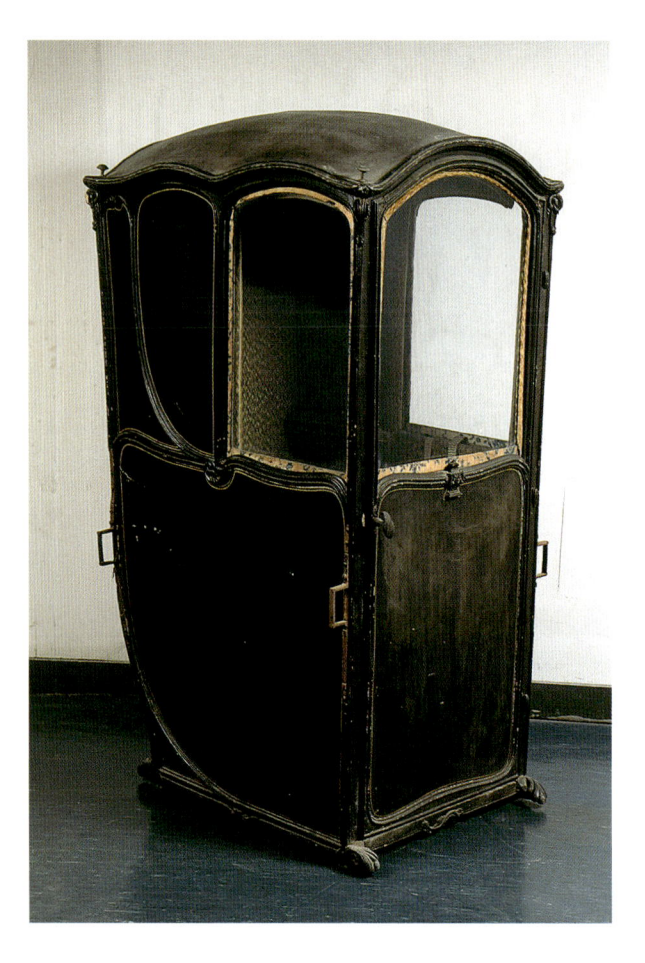

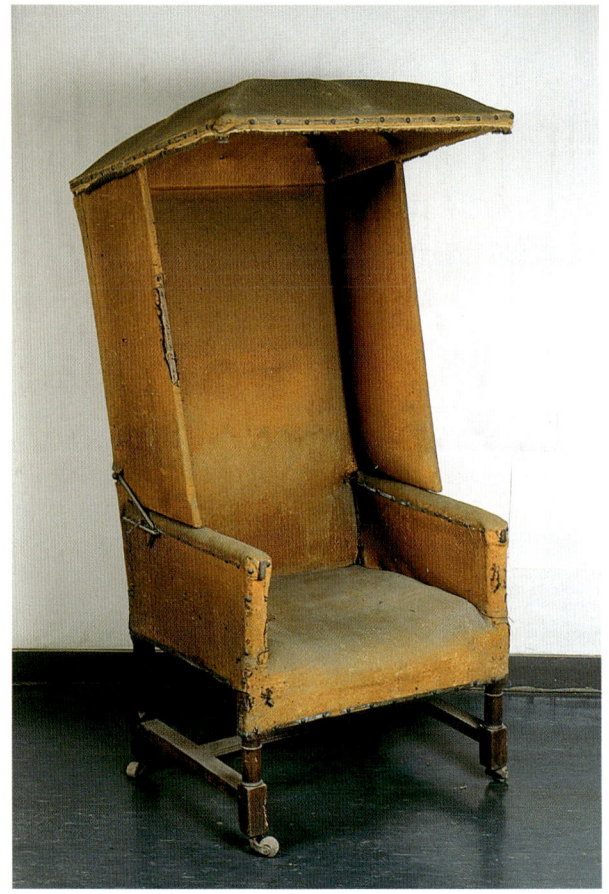

A curious kind of chair known as a *guérite* had wheels, an adjustable rack and pinion back, a hinged canopy and two sliding rods in the armrests for holding a tray.
Other interesting items were the furnishings for the hospital's administrative section: the boardroom contained a large table and sets of high-quality chairs and armchairs.

The dove tapestries

Among the "property, furniture and other things presently belonging to the great hospital of Beaune", the 1501 inventory mentions "thirty-one *haute lisse* coverings with a dove pattern". At the time *haute lisse* referred not to the vertical weaving technique but to the superior quality of the tapestries laid on the beds in the Great Hall on feast days. Almost identical, they have a marbled red background on which the chancellor's motto "Alone", followed by a star, alternates with a row of doves perched on broken branches amid the entwined initials of the founders. At the centre and in the corners shields hanging from the largest branches bear Guigone de Salins' coat of arms: on an azure ground, the three keys of the Rolin family and the castellated tower of the Salins. This kind of tapestry was not uncommon in the Middle Ages: the coat of arms identified the person commissioning the work – who in this case was also the female donor.
Among the numerous cushions, the inventory mentions "six handsome squares bearing the arms of the founders", which may be the source of the two fragments kept at the Hôtel-Dieu. One shows the shield with the chancellor's three golden keys set on a background that includes wavy leaves. On the other his wife's coat of arms, surrounded by the motto "Alone" and the star, is set among oak branches arranged in the shape of a diamond.

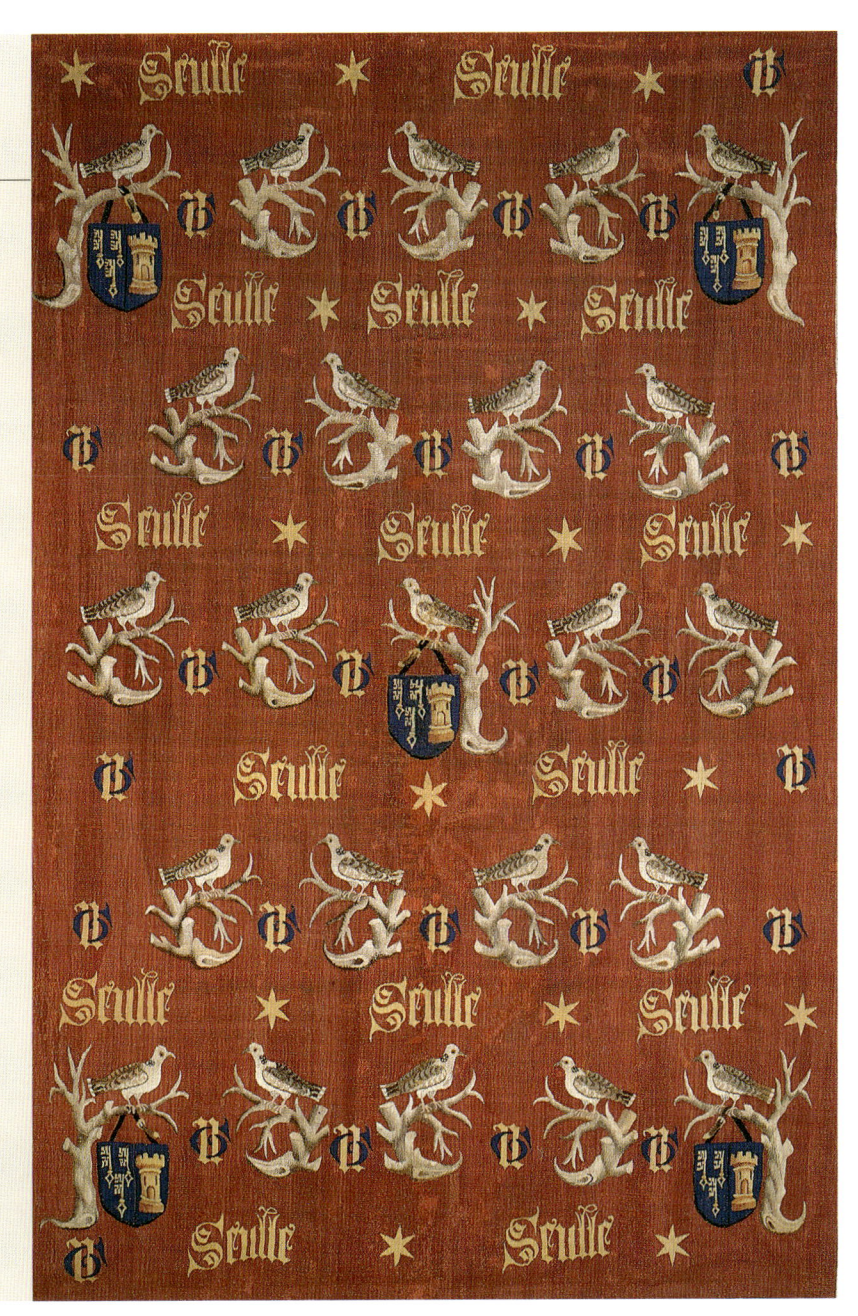

Everyday items

■ Below: *Cleaning Copperware in the Hôtel-Dieu Courtyard*, watercolour by Émile Goussery, 1933.
Facing page: Pewterware.

The everyday running of the hospital called for all sorts of objects relating to food and medical care. Daily use meant, of course, wear and tear and regular replacement of these items. The Hôtel-Dieu's substantial surviving stock of copper and brass kitchen utensils mostly dates from the 18th and 19th centuries. In a 1933 painting from the life the Beaune artist Émile Goussery showed the nuns polishing up their kitchen equipment.

In the 15th century monasteries, convents and hospitals began using pewter for their tableware, a practice that often lasted into the early 20th century, even though the much cheaper earthenware had already been available for more than a hundred years. In the 19th century pewterers were fewer and fewer and made only everyday and medical items.

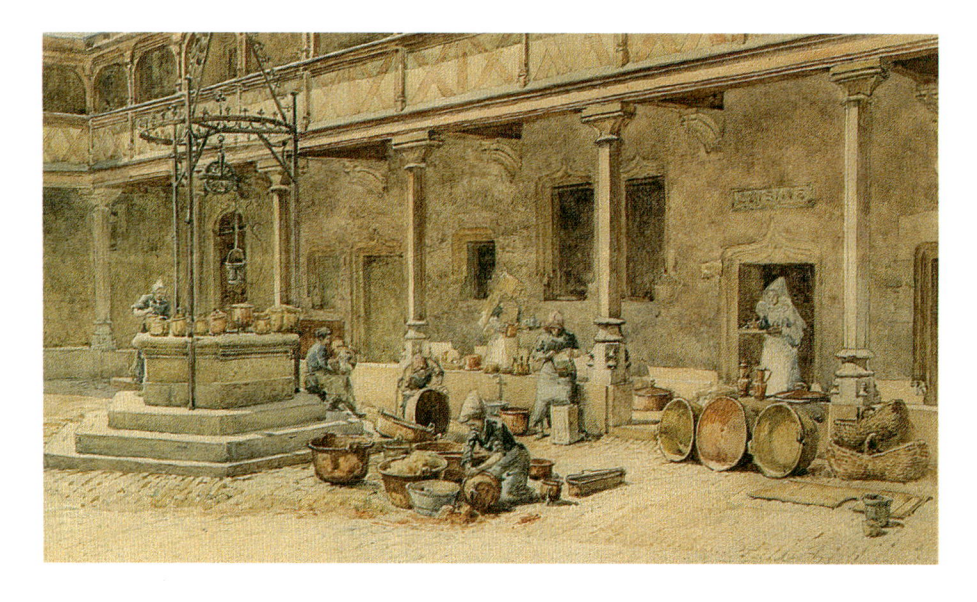

No pewterware earlier than the 17th century has survived at the Hôtel-Dieu, as the practice of casting allowed for the making of new pieces by melting down old, damaged ones. Mention was made in 1501 of an attic containing "twenty pounds of broken pewter" waiting to be reused; and in 1793 it was noted that the number of pewter pieces for the patients was being steadily reduced "by the melting down and casting that was necessary from time to time". It was then decided to transfer the nuns' pewterware to the patients and offer the good sisters earthenware crockery.

As is to be expected, the commonest items had to do with food and medical care, these being the hospital's primary concerns: porringers, plates, jugs, tumblers, bleeding basins, hot-water bottles and various types of syringe. Almost all of them were marked with a shield bearing the letters IHS, Christ's monogram: the matrices for the stamp – one from the 18th and one from the 19th century – can still be seen at the Hôtel-Dieu.

The hospital obtained its supplies from pewterers in Beaune and Dijon, but many locally made everyday items carry no maker's mark. The few pieces from elsewhere are certainly donations: a ewer from Bern in Switzerland, a pharmacy jar by L.M.P. Favre of Lyon and a wall stoup whose flower-decorated cross is held by two cherubs. Many Beaune pewterers worked for the Hôtel-Dieu in the 17th and 18th centuries, and if no trace remains there of the output of such local dynasties as the Dominos, Amelines and Riolons, it is doubtless because of the recycling of worn-out items.

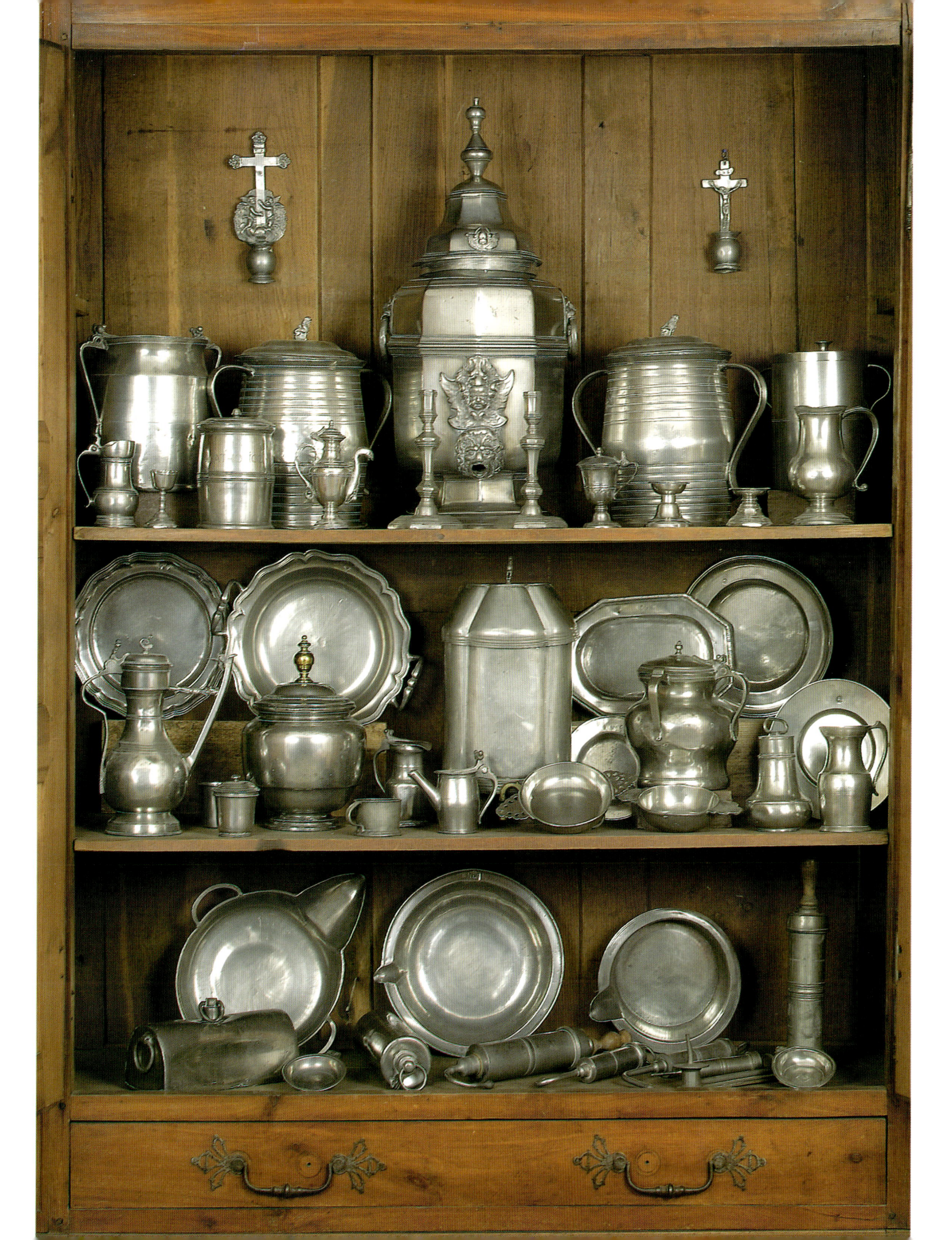

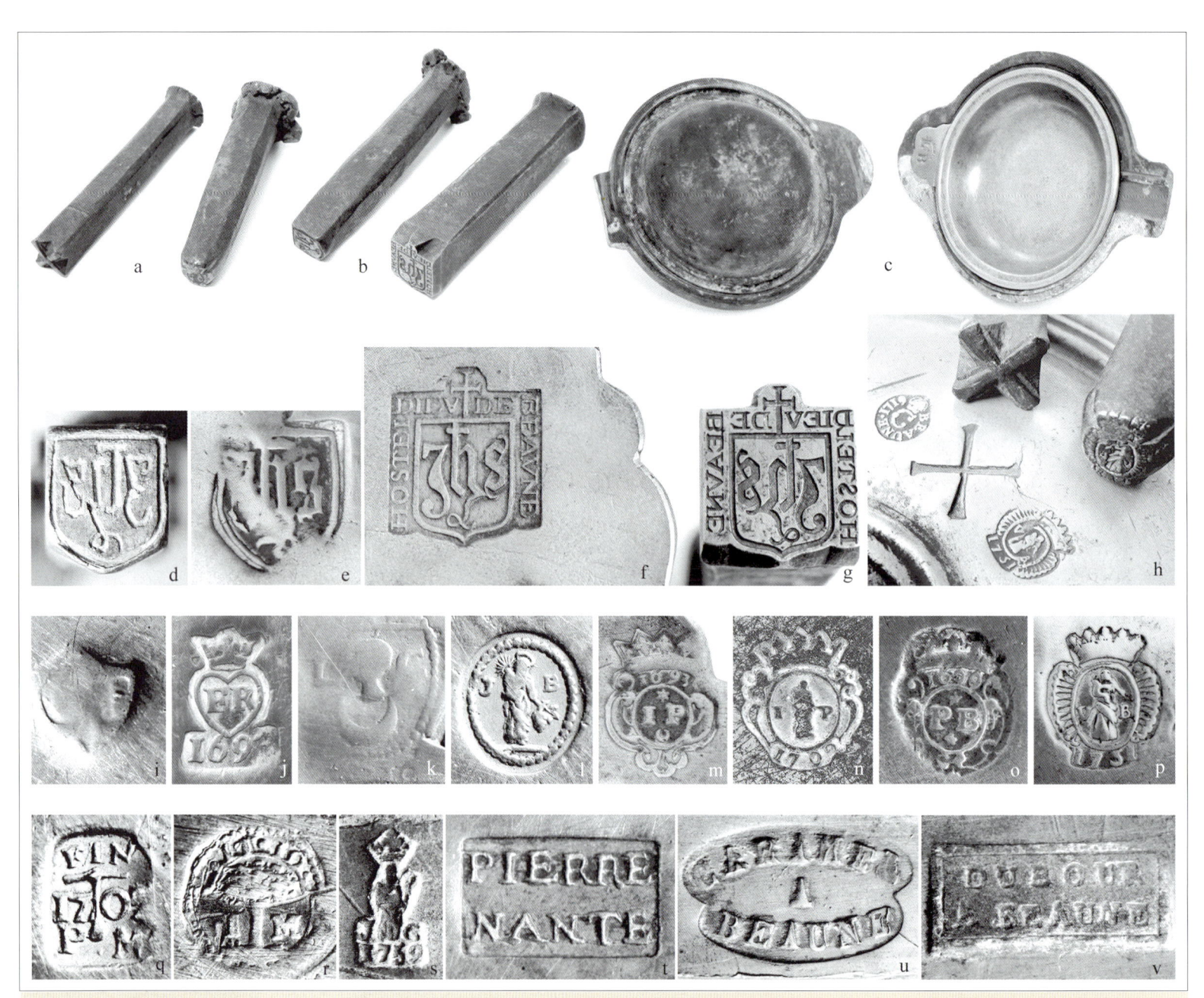

A selection of pewter stamps:

a. Matrices for the stamps of pewterer Vivant Bornier.
b. Matrices for Hôtel-Dieu property stamps: one 17th century, the other 19th century.
c. A bleeding bowl in its mould.
d., e. Hôtel-Dieu property matrix and stamp, 17th century.
f., g. Hôtel-Dieu property matrix and stamp, 19th century.
h. Matrices and stamps of pewterer Vivant Bornier.

Stamps of pewterers who worked for the Hôtel-Dieu:

i. C. F: Claude Forest, from Beaune, mentioned from 1643 to 1683.
j. F. R. 1693: François Routy the Younger, born in Beaune in 1663, master craftsman in 1687, mentioned until 1703.
k. L. C. 1710(?): Louis Chenu, from Beaune, married in 1716, mentioned until 1729.
l. J. B.: Jean Bouzereau, from Beaune, first mentioned 1698, died 1758.
m., n. I. P. 1693 and I.P. 1702: Jean Parigot the Younger, from Beaune, master craftsman in 1687, mentioned until 1707.
o. P. B. 1699: Philibert Bornier, from Beaune, born c. 1673, master craftsman in 1699, died 1738.
p. V. B. 1751: Vivant Bornier, from Beaune, born 1703, died 1765.
q. P. M. 1702: Fine pewterware stamp of Paul Mutinot(?), from Dijon, born c. 1645, master craftsman in 1680, died 1726.
r. I. M. 1710: Jacques Mousseau, from Dijon, born c. 1674, master craftsman in 1710, died 1721.
s. I. G. 1759: Jean-Joseph Guyot, from Dijon, born 1729, master craftsman in 1759, died 1766.
t. Pierre Nante, worked in Beaune 1796–99.
u. Caramel à Beaune: Thomas Caramello, born in Varzo (Piedmont) 1775, married in Beaune in 1844 and again in 1852, at which time he left the city.
v. Dubour à Beaune: Barthelemi Borca, born in Tapia (Piedmont) 1775, married Thérèse, daughter of pewterer Jean-Baptiste Bornier in 1803, changed his name to Dubour, died 1860.

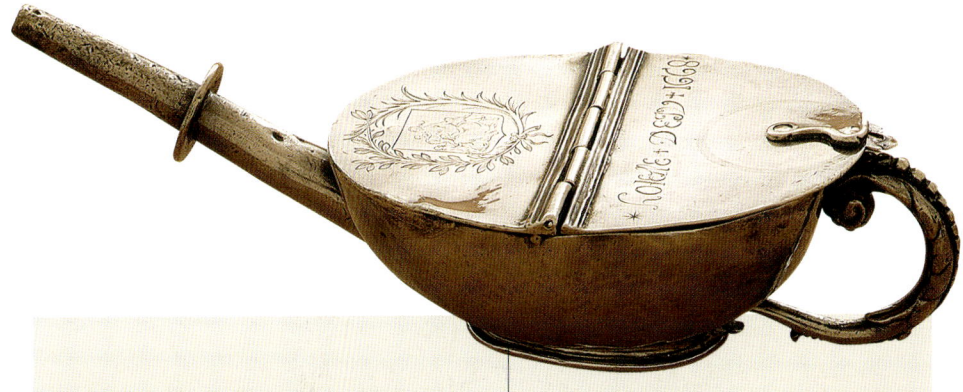

The only surviving pieces are a few bowls and bleeding basins bearing the marks of Claude Forest, who worked between 1643 and 1683; François Routy, son and brother of pewterers, who became a master-pewterer in 1687; Louis Chenu, mentioned in the parish registers for 1716-29; and Jean Bouzereau, who in 1698 worked with Philibert Bornier on repairs to the roof of the Great Hall. Son and father of pewterers, Jean Parigot, made a master craftsman in 1687, was the creator of pieces that included two medicine pots; in 1699 the Hôtel-Dieu provided him with moulds and other equipment.

The Borniers cast a pair of torches, one stamped with the name of Philibert, made a master craftsman in 1699, and the other with that of his son Vivant. The latter made a series of flour containers in the shape of hooped kegs, with a seated lion on the lids: the poor-house hospice had one of these, but bearing Philibert Bornier's stamp – being expensive, the moulds were handed down from father to son.

There is no documentary reference to a resident pewterer at the Hôtel-Dieu, yet it seems that Vivant Bornier held this post and worked in the hospital: the matrix for his stamp, dated 1751, remained there after him. Usually the matrix was destroyed when its owner ceased work.

A preserves container is the sole surviving work by Pierre Nante, otherwise known in Beaune only for the payment of a trade tax in 1796-99.

The hospital also possesses items by the 18th-century Dijon pewterers Paul Mutinot, Jacques Mousseau and Jean-Joseph Guyot, who became master craftsmen in, respectively, 1680, 1710 and 1759.

Beaune's two 19th-century pewterers were Italians: Thomas Caramello – or Caramel – left the city in 1852, and Barthelemi Borca, known as Dubour, came to live there after his marriage to Thérèse Bornier. Both mainly made basins, fountains and enema syringes.

Bianchi, a pewterer active in Dijon in the mid-19th century, was the last practitioner of the trade to work for the Hôtel-Dieu. He worked in the hospital and the moulds he used for his jugs, tumblers, bowls with handles and bleeding bowls have survived. He also made flour containers and cylindrical hot-water bottles.

A rare hospital feeding cup

An everyday item in the hospitals of the time, the feeding cup was usually made of pewter or earthenware. The inscription on this one – *Hotelle + Deiu + 1668* – clearly indicates who it belongs to. More than just a rare example of 17th-century civic silverware, it combines a functional shape with especially sophisticated decoration: the base of the neck is encircled with applied ornament, the handle is decorated with scrolled foliage highlighted with pearls, and a shield bearing an allegory of charity is engraved on the fixed part of the lid. The stamps are those of the Beaune silversmith Philibert Viénot – a proof of high-quality local workmanship that only adds to the interest of the piece.

From hospital to museum

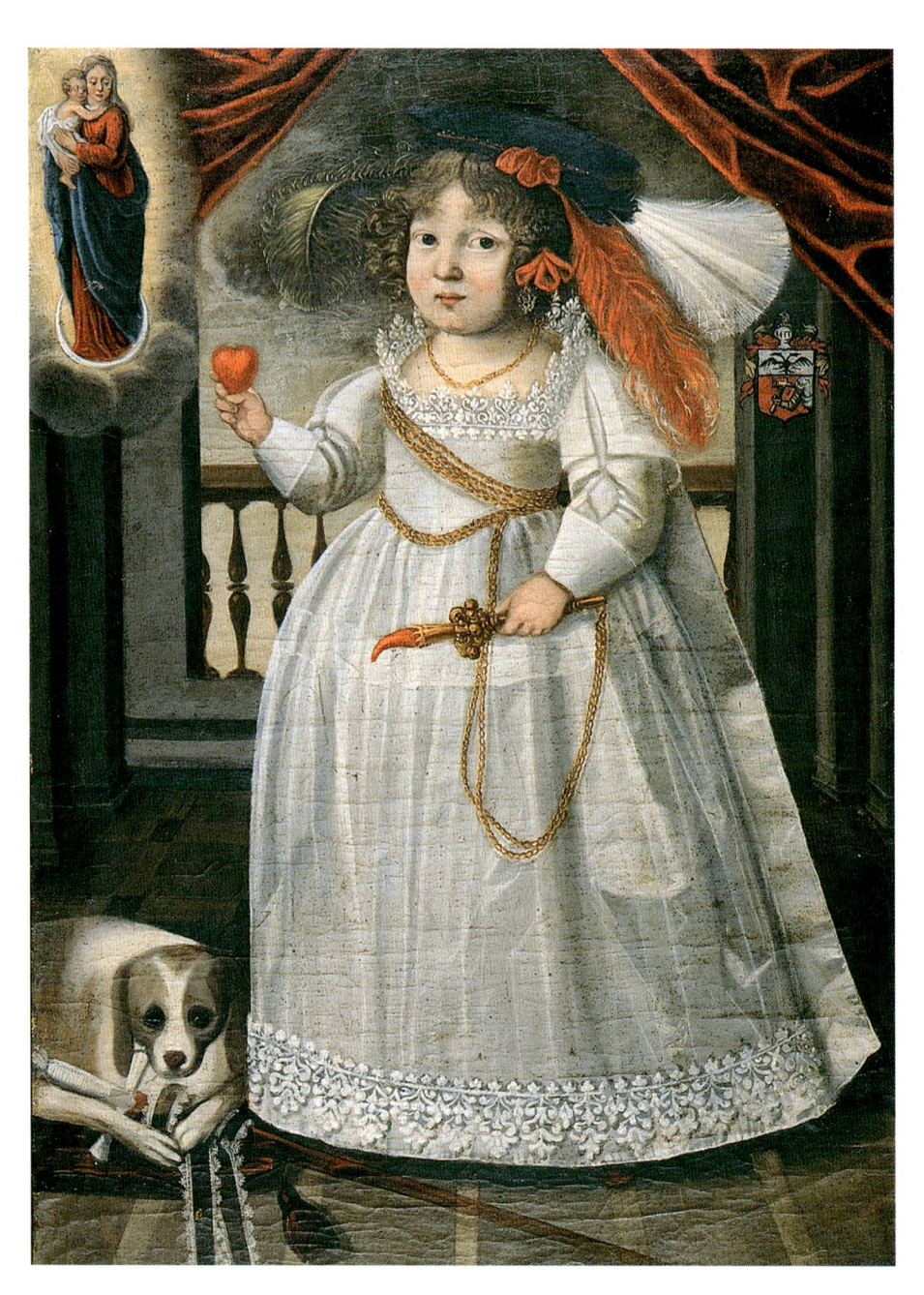

As its archives indicate, the Hôtel-Dieu has been the recipient of gifts and legacies from benefactors and patients from the very beginning down to the present day: houses, estates, vineyards, meadow and farmland, sums of money, furniture, crockery and linen. To the original furniture were added handsome cupboards, carved chests, chairs and armchairs in a wide range of styles, together with statues, paintings, tapestries and all sorts of miscellaneous objects. The collection – half of it furniture – now comprises some five thousand items.

Some of these pieces relate to benefactors, like the moving portrait of Catherine, daughter of Jean Massol, who died when still a child. She is shown wearing a dress of white satin edged with lace and an extravagant hat with red and white feathers. The gesture with which she offers her heart to the Virgin is somewhat conventional, but the rattle in her left hand and the little dog lying at her feet give this work a touching grace.

AN IMPRESSIVE TAPESTRY COLLECTION

The original tapestries were the beginning of the remarkable collection built up over the centuries. Bequests, purchases, commissions and donations have added Flemish and Aubusson examples dating from the early 16th to the late 18th century.

On its old lining the "mille fleurs" tapestry of St Eligius (*Fr.* Saint-Éloi) was marked "Parizot", the name of an old Beaune family, one of whose members became a nun at the Hôtel-Dieu. Made up of a number of arbitrarily assembled pieces dating from the early 16th century, the tapestry shows, to the right, St Fiacre, patron saint of gardeners; to the left, a seated lady; and in the centre, kneeling before the Virgin, a horseman holding the bridle of a horse with one leg missing. Only this third figure

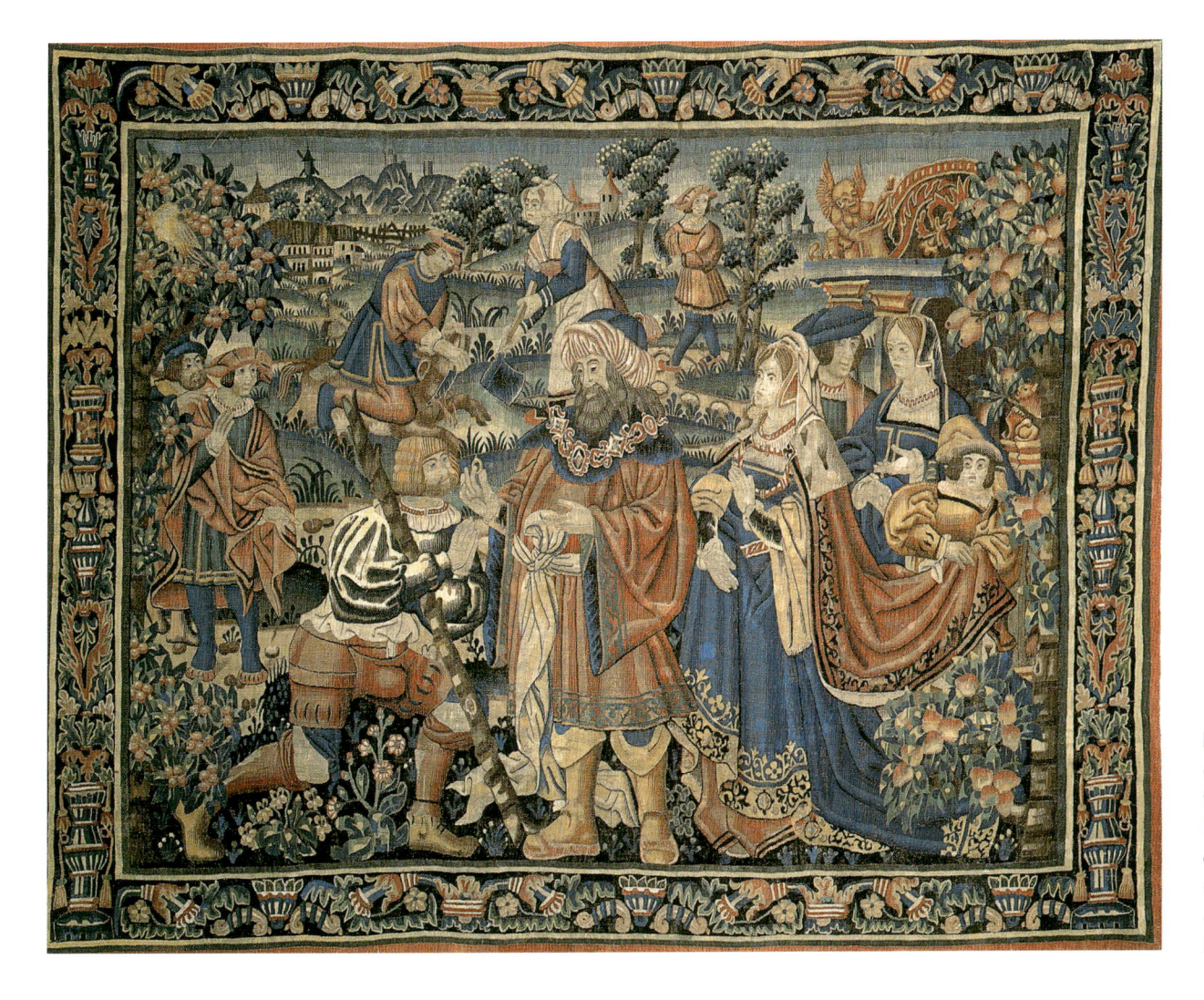

▌Facing page: Portrait of Catherine de Massol, first half 17th century. Left: *Return of the Prodigal Son*, early 16th century, listed as a historical monument in 1943.

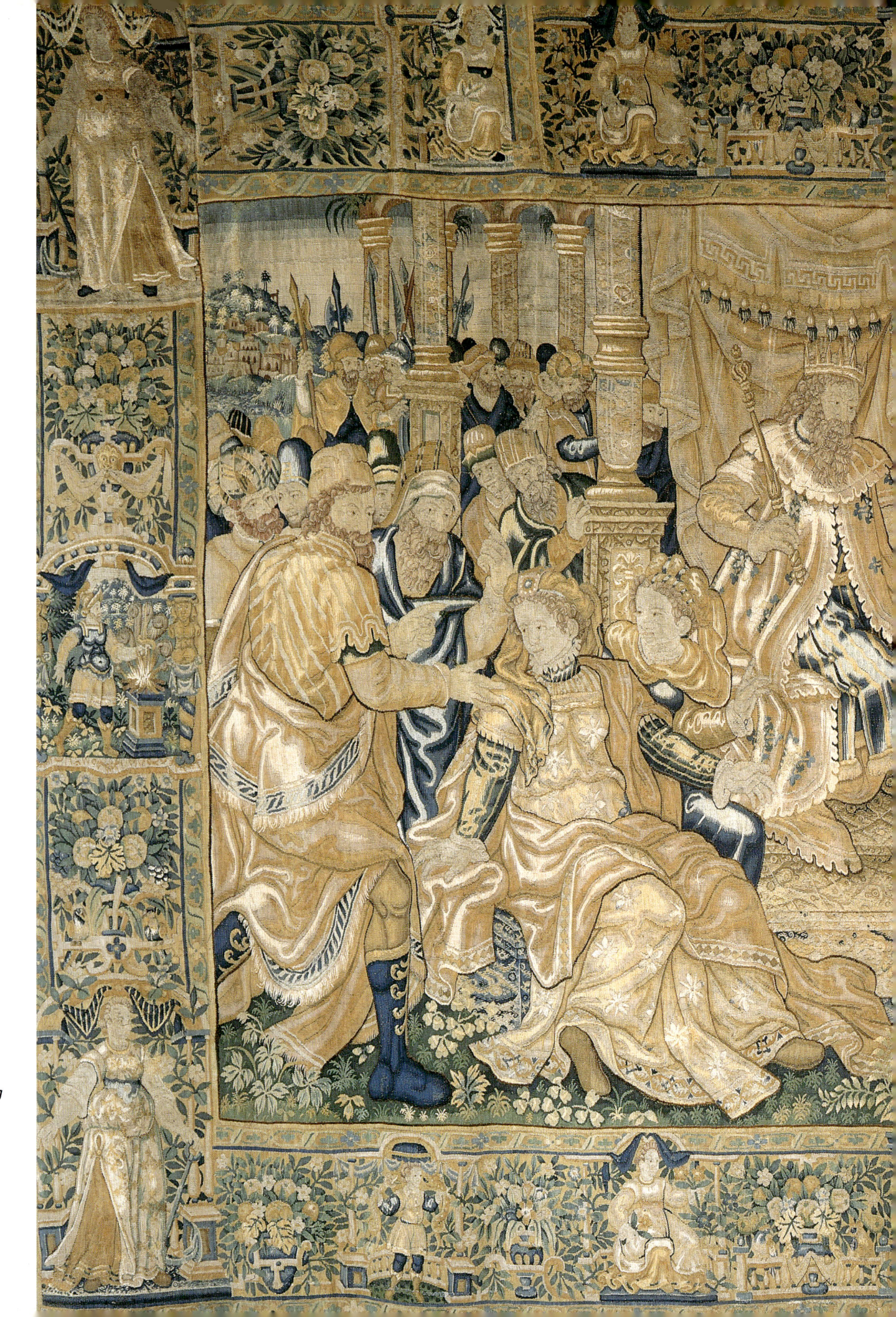

▌ Right: *David Learning of the Death of Absalom*, Audenarde tapestry, late 16th century.

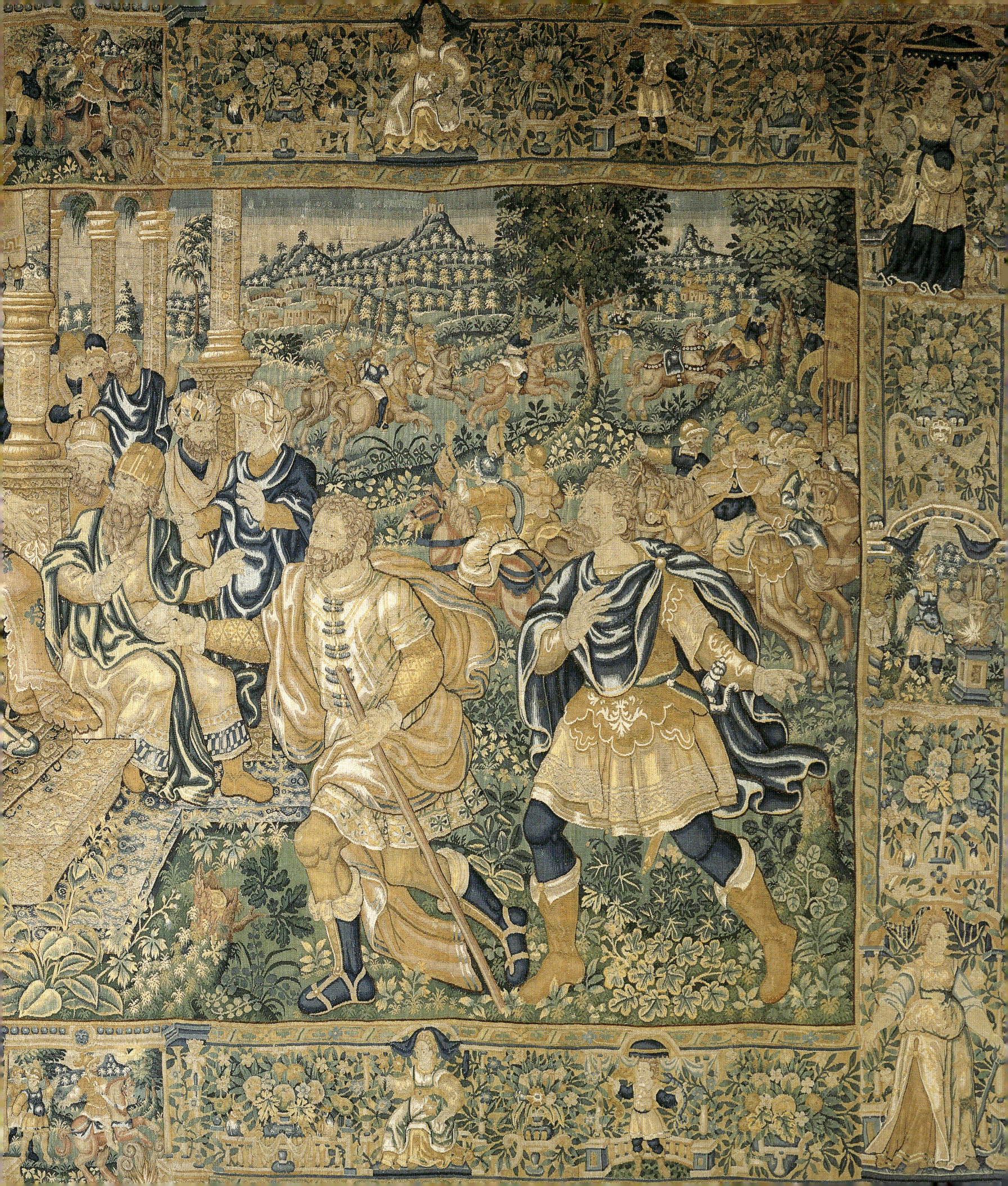

■ Above: *The legend of St Eligius*, mille fleurs tapestry, early 16th century, listed as a historical monument in 1944.
Facing page:
Below left: *The Blessing of Jacob*, Brussels tapestry, early 17th century.
Below right: *Diana Bathing*, Aubusson tapestry, second half 16th century.

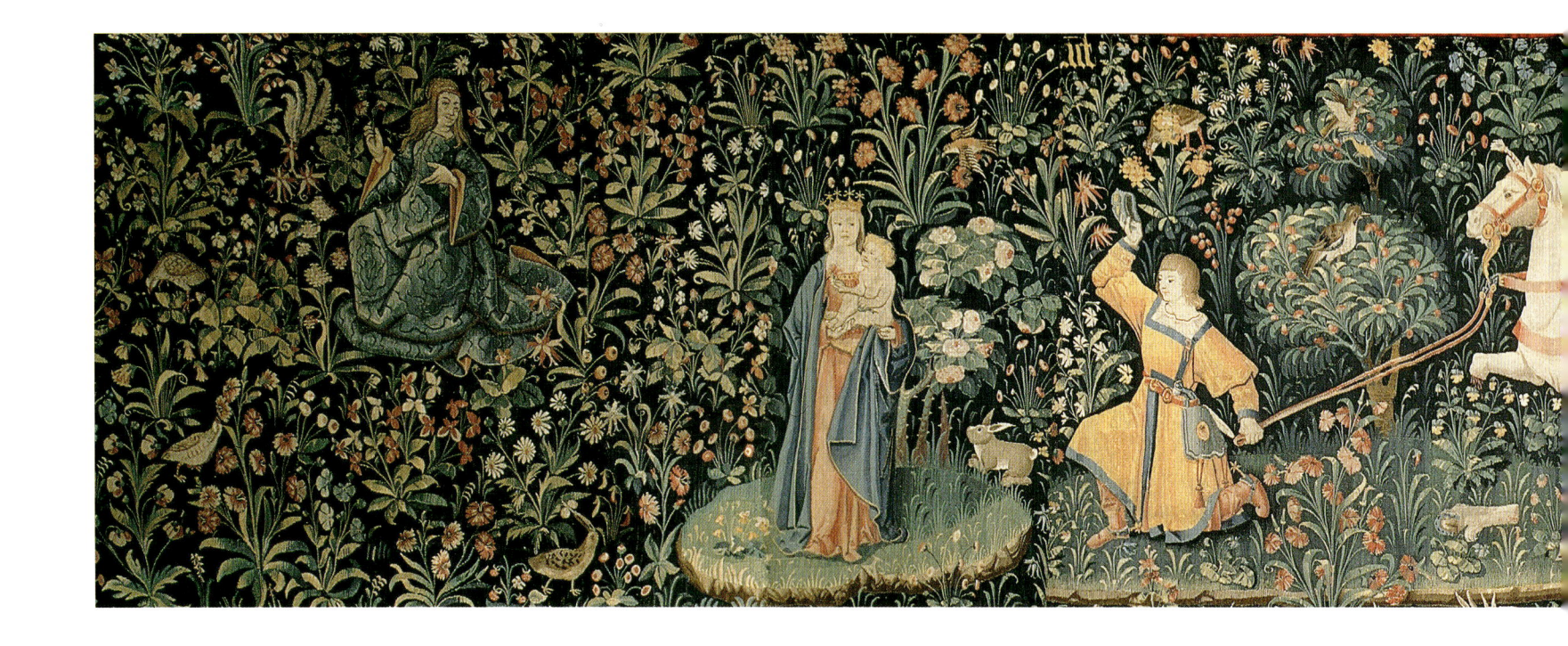

actually belongs to the legend of St Eligius, whose name is woven in at several points. Despite its fragmentary nature, the work retains a certain unity thanks to its navy blue background dotted with flowers, rabbits and birds.

The *Prodigal Son* hanging – this was a popular subject in the 16th century – was in fact an excuse for a portrayal of the leisure activities of the ruling classes. Of its seven sections only the last two really relate to the biblical parable: *The Prodigal Son Feeding Swine* and *The Return of the Prodigal Son*. Their style indicates the source of these Flemish tapestries as the workshops at Tournai.

Attributed to the Audenarde workshops, a handsome late 16th-century tapestry shows King David learning of the death of his son Absalom. The wide borders with their mingling of allegorical figures and little mythological scenes, some set beneath a "pergola" and each separated from its neighbour by bouquets of flowers and fruit, are characteristic of the Flemish output of the time.

In 1749 the Hôtel-Dieu acquired from a Paris dealer a five-piece *Story of Jacob* bearing the mark of Brussels weaver Martin Reymbouts. This group of tapestries was woven in the early 17th century from cartoons based on drawings by the painter Bernard Van Orley, also from Brussels.

Another biblical theme, the sacrifice of Abraham, is the subject of a tapestry identifiable as an Aubusson by the mark on its lower hem. This 17th-century piece was commissioned by the Hôtel-Dieu, whose coat of arms is woven into the upper border.

Mythology is represented by two late 17th-century Aubusson works recounting the story of Achilles and another of Diana bathing. Their model may have been cartoons prepared by the painter Isaac Moillon, active in the region in the 1660s.

In 1897 five framed tapestries came to brighten up the board of directors' office. Against a landscape background we see suitors murmuring sweet nothings to shepherdesses as other young people entertain themselves innocently, notably with archery and games of blind man's buff. Drawn from paintings of pastoral scenes and village festivals, these subjects were much appreciated in the second half of the 18th century.

111

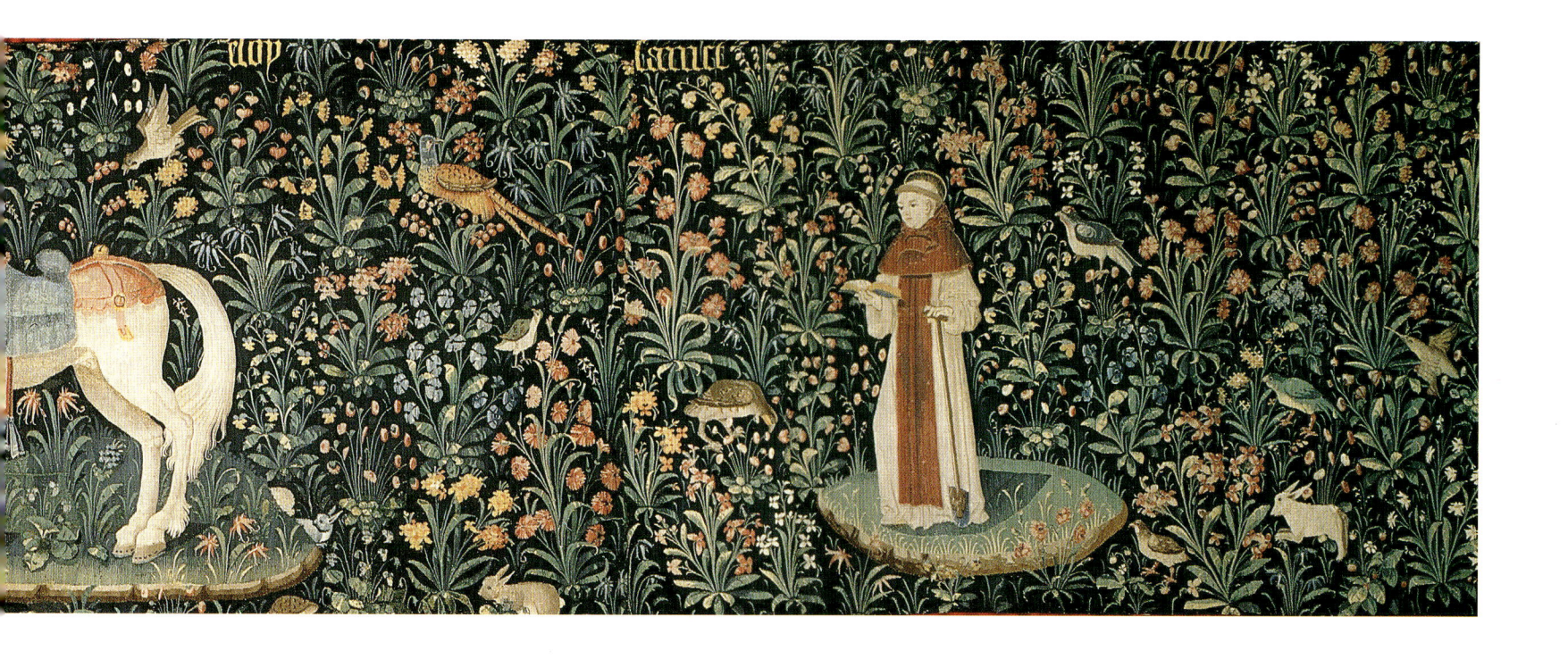

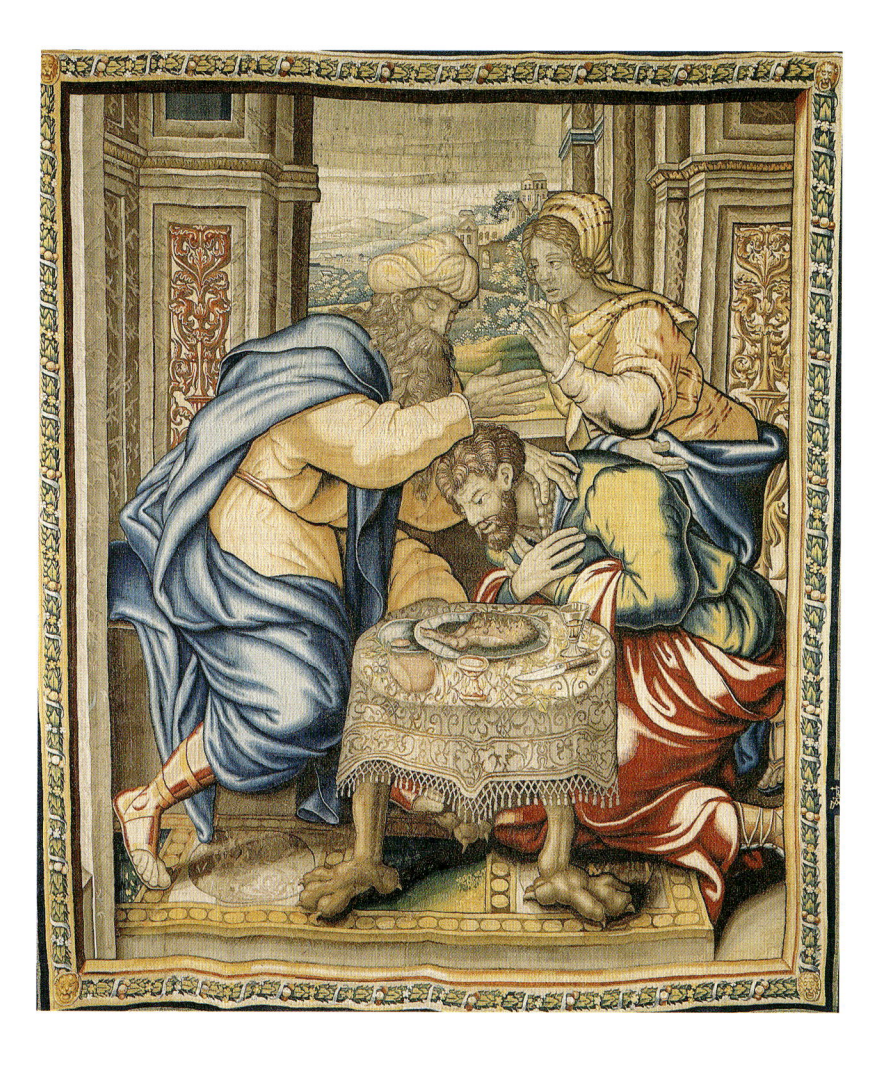

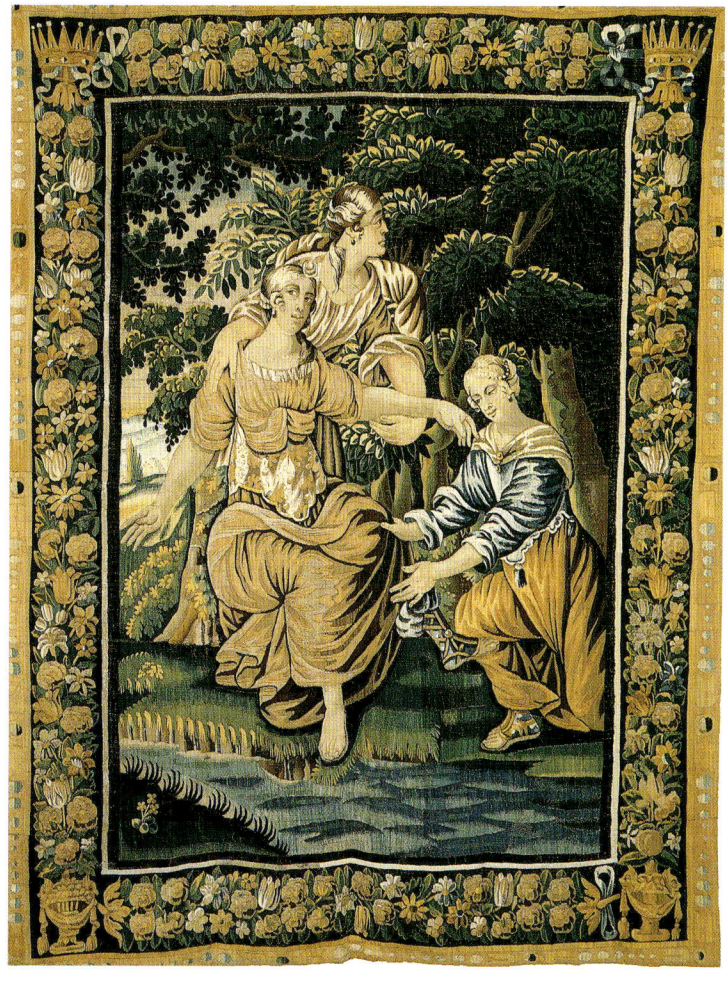

■ Right: *The Sacrifice of Abraham*, Aubusson tapestry, 16th century.

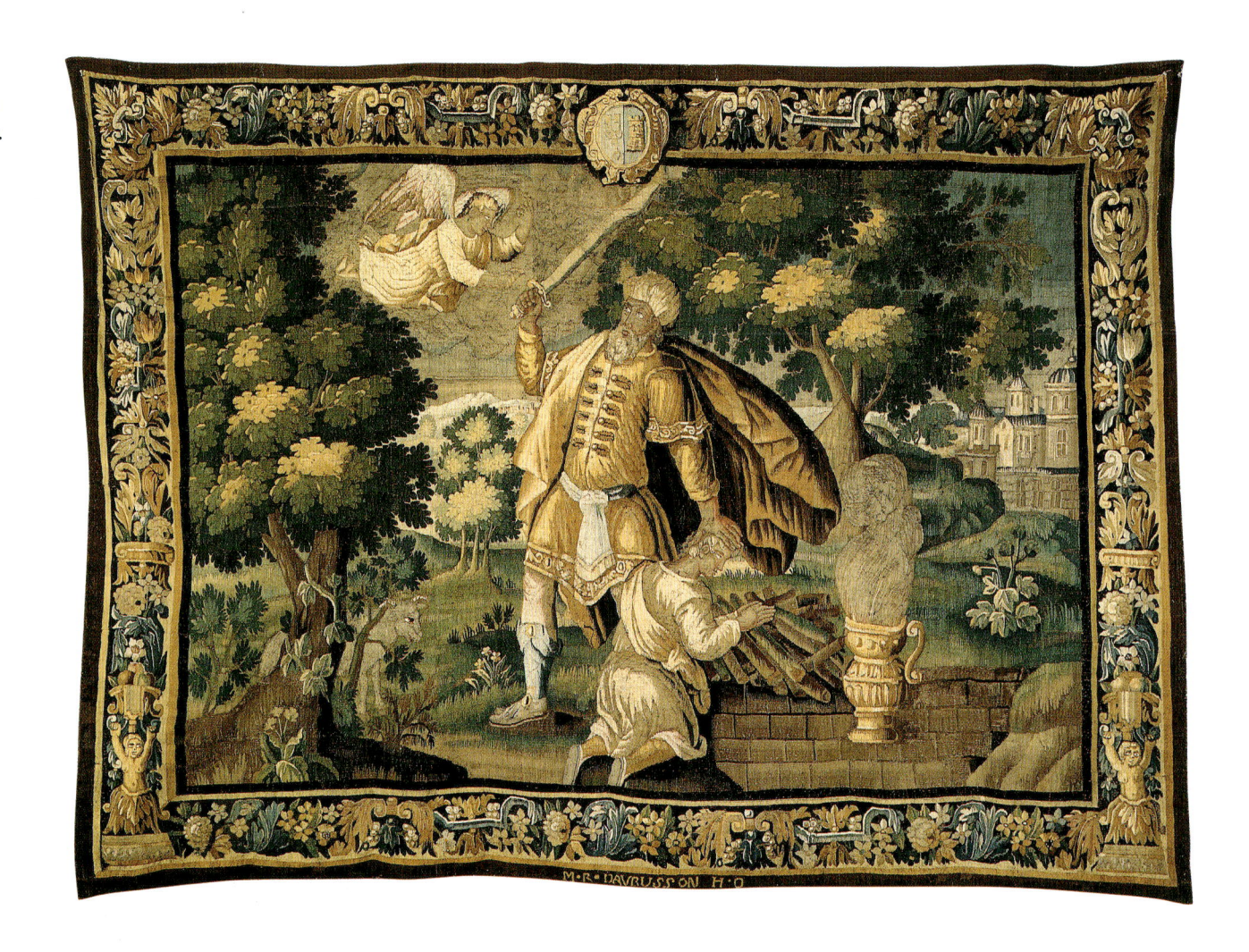

The Hôtel-Dieu collection also includes many "verdures" in the Flemish and Aubusson styles. The oldest of these, from the southern Low Countries, are characterised by luxuriant vegetation and broad, opulent borders: the large stag tapestry is a typical example of the genre.

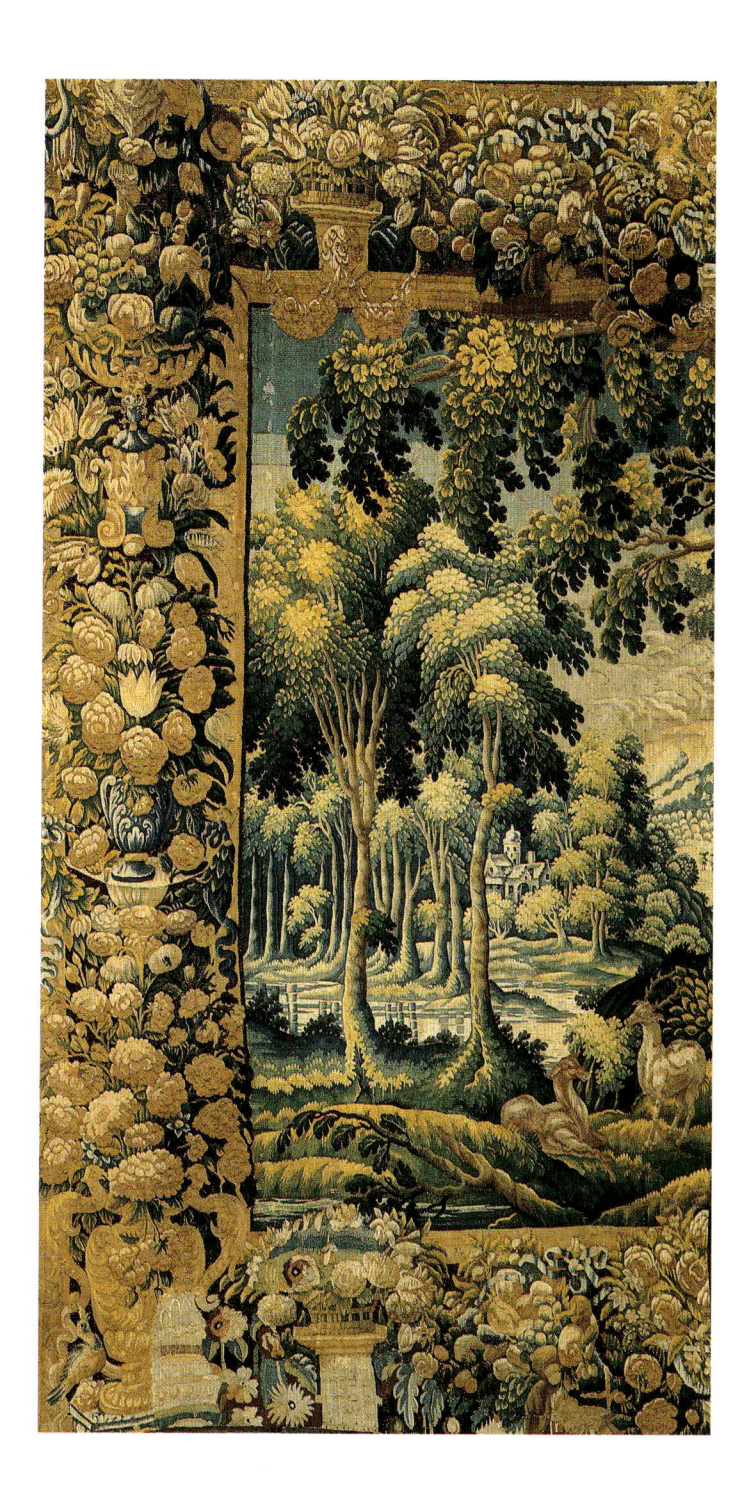

■ Above: Large stag tapestry (detail), Flanders, 17th century.
Above right: Decorated casket, 15th century, listed as a historical monument in 1944.

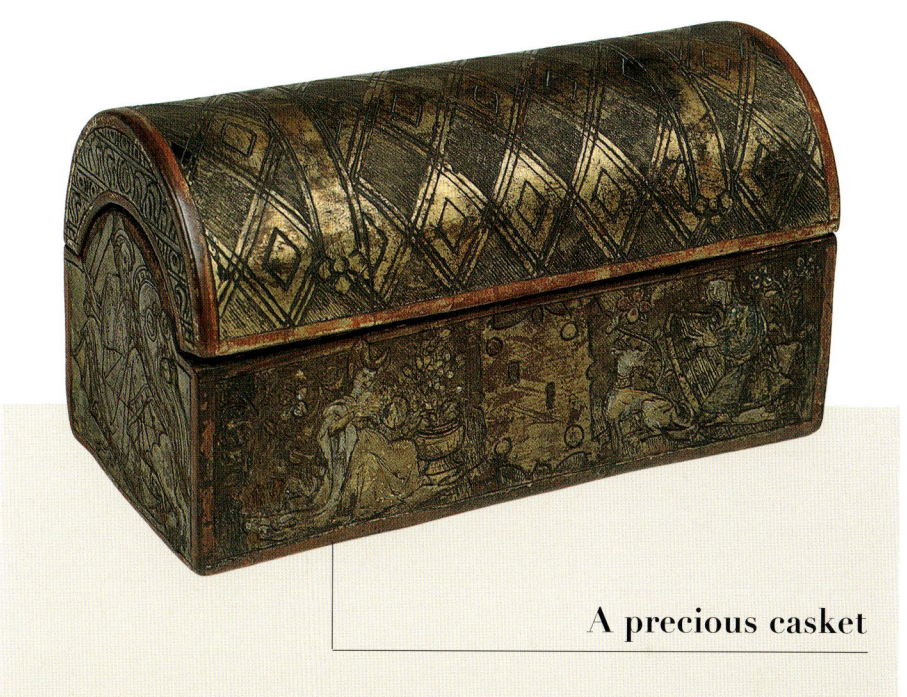

A precious casket

The work of a "master casemaker and chest dresser", this casket of fruit-tree wood with its rounded lid is entirely covered with fine, pliant leather. Red on the inside, it is for the most part gilded, with coloured highlights, on the outside. It has no lock or metal reinforcement, but these features have been simulated with a scriber. The lid is decorated with a diamond pattern and the underside of the casket with a fleur de lys. On each side is a grotesque human figure, one making music with a bellows and poker, the other holding a shield that shows a bearded, bespectacled face with a protruding tongue. On the back, flanked by two mythical beasts, is the scene from the *Roman de Renart* in which Reynard the Fox preaches to Chantecleer the Cock and his hens. The front bears a scene of courtly love: to one side of the false lock a lady is weaving a wreath, while to the other a young man with a dog is playing the harp.

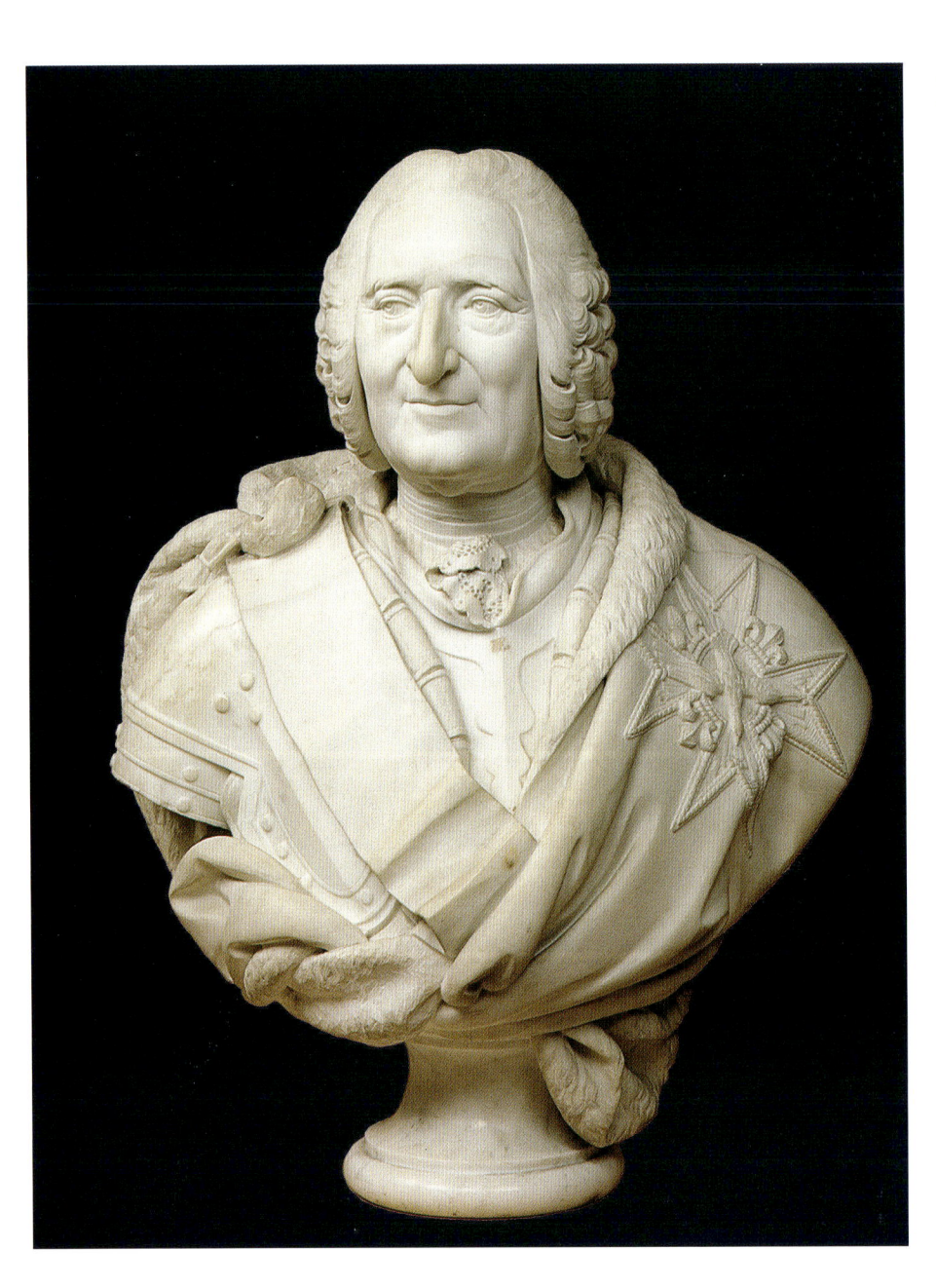

A SOUVENIR OF THE CLERMONT-TONNERRE FAMILY

In 1981 Prince Florent de Mérode donated to the Hospices de Beaune a number of works belonging to the Clermont-Tonnerre family. As descendents of the Rolins, several members of the family had held the title of temporal patron of the Hôtel-Dieu.

Created in 1767 by the royal sculptor Augustin Pajou, the handsome bust in veined white marble of Gaspard de Clermont-Tonnerre was exhibited at the Salon in Paris in the same year. It shows the marquess, then seventy nine, at the end of a brilliant career culminating in the rank of marshal of France. Sporting the *bigotière* wig of a former officer, he wears the sash of a knight of the Order of the Holy Spirit over his breastplate and the order's insignia on his cloak. The sculptor has brought great subtlety and skill to his rendering of the different fabrics and other materials. Gaspard's younger son, Monsignor Anne-Antoine-Jules de Clermont-Tonnerre was invited in 1816 to assume the patronage of the Hôtel-Dieu, but preferred to renounce his ancient family rights. His portrait by Louis Hersent, a much sought-after painter under the Restoration and the July Monarchy, dates from 1827.

The Hôtel-Dieu also holds the prelate's two sets of silver-gilt ornaments and plate, the first of which dates from his time as bishop of Châlons-en-

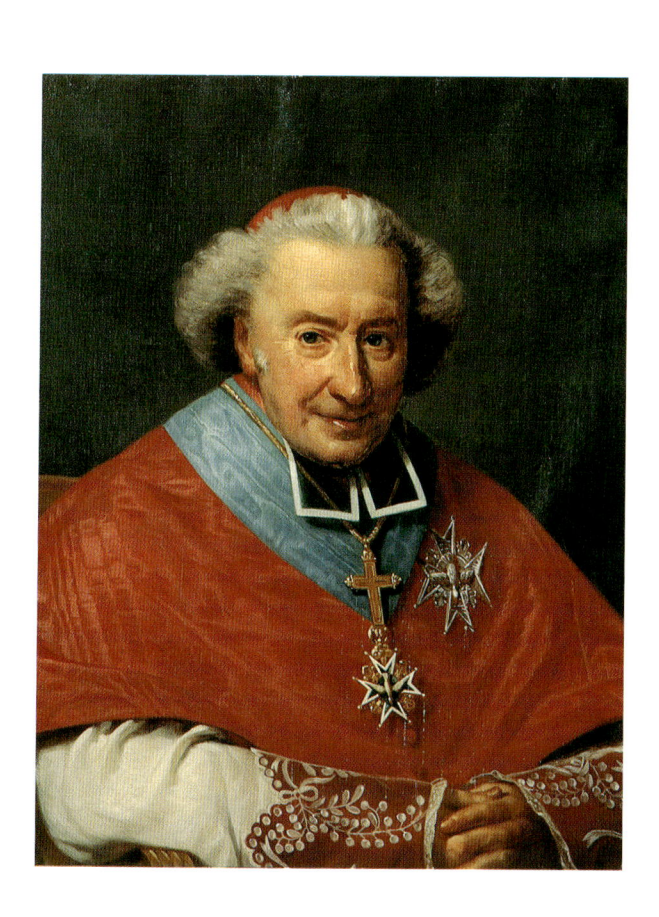

Champagne. The work of Strasbourg goldsmith Jean-Geoffroy Fritz in 1789-90, it consists of eight silver items bearing no decoration. The second, from after the Revolution, was made by Paris goldsmith Edme Gelez when its owner was archbishop of Toulouse: each piece was engraved with his coat of arms after he was made a cardinal in 1822. More extensive and above all more ornate than its predecessor, this set is still kept in its original black leather-covered chest.

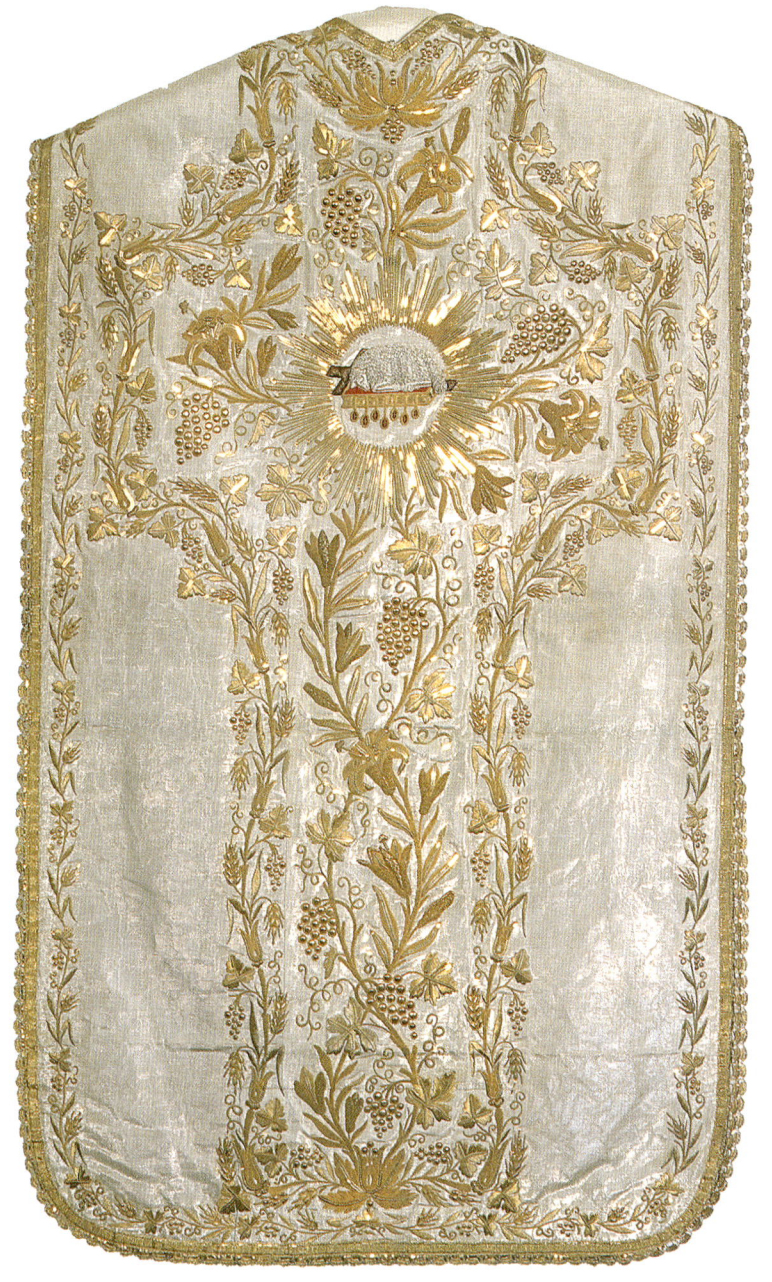

▌ Previous pages:
Left: Bust of Gaspard de Clermont-Tonnerre by Augustin Pajou, 1767.
Right: Portrait of Cardinal de Clermont-Tonnerre by Louis Hersent, 1827.
Far right: Chasuble, early 19th century.
Right: Bishop's altar-plate (partial view), made by Jean-Geoffroy Fritz in 1789-90.
Facing page: Bishop's altar-plate, made by Edme Gelez between 1812-27.

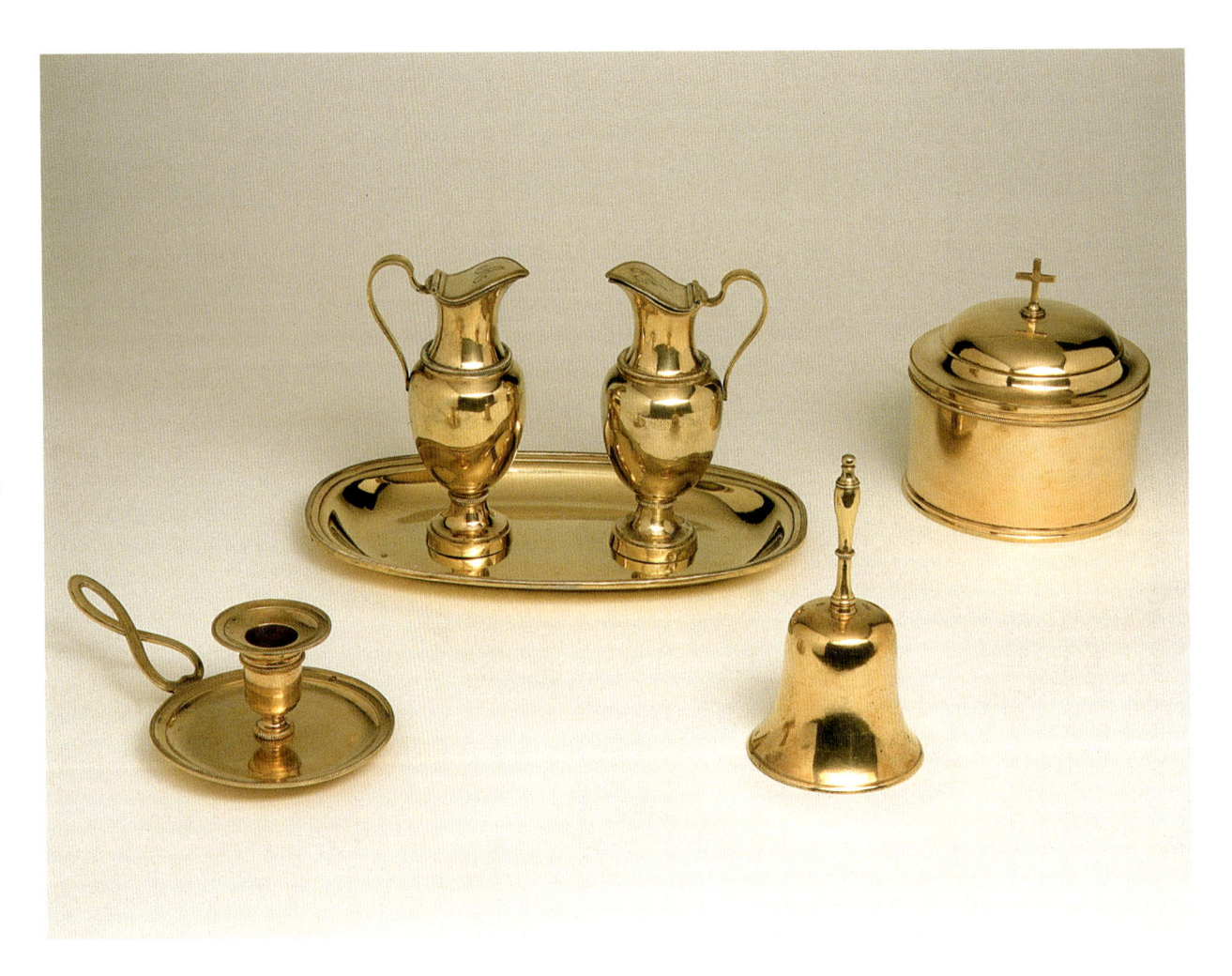

The elaborately engraved and embossed decoration is in the Neoclassical goldsmithing style of the period; in many respects it resembles that of the ornaments and plate commissioned from the same craftsman by the Duchesse de Berry and now in the Dobrée Museum in Nantes.

The cardinal's vestments were also included in the donation: embroidered chasubles with their accessories, tunicles, mitres, sandals and gloves are fine examples of Catholic ritual apparel from the first third of the 19th century.

116

117

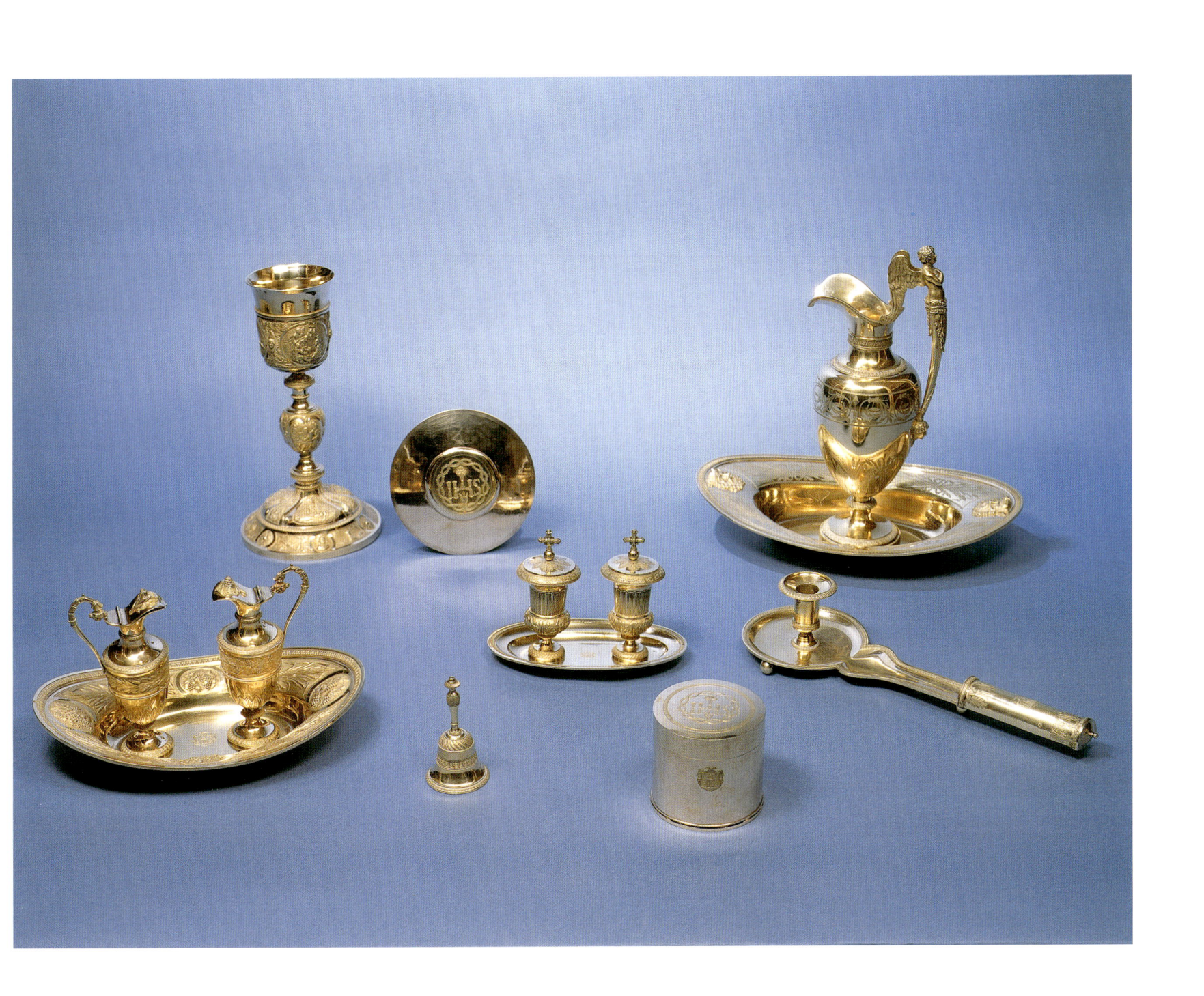

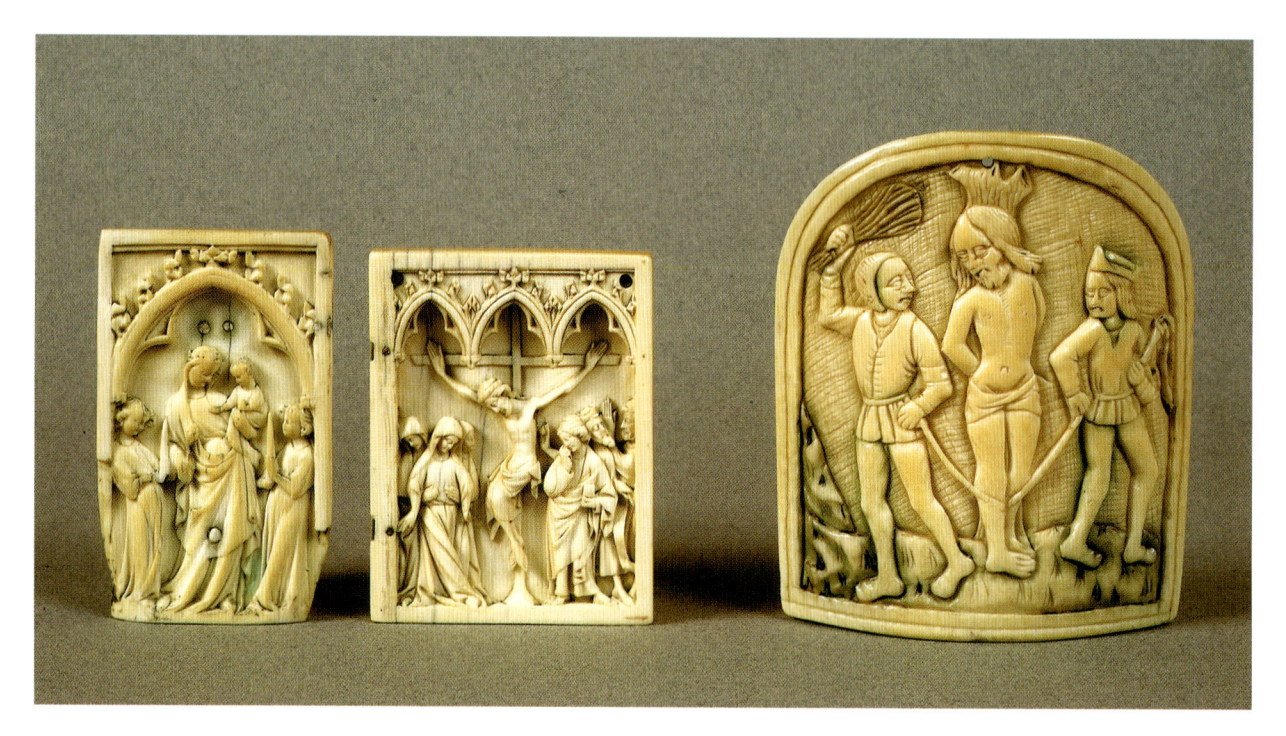

■ Right: Ivory plaques and osculatorium, listed as historical monuments in 1944.
Below: Wine-tasting cup made by Gaspard Simonnot in 1754.

THE BEQUEST OF A DISCERNING COLLECTOR

A lover of art and archaeology, the Dijon architect Albert Humbert built up a collection of objets d'art, antique furniture, paintings, books, sculpture, stained glass and carved ivory. As the son of a Beaune goldsmith, it seemed to him natural to make the Hôtel-Dieu his sole heir in 1884. After his death in 1892, the additions to the hospital collection included a rare ivory osculatorium showing the flagellation of Christ from the late 15th century, some small 14th-century ivory tablets carved with images of a Crucifixion and the Virgin and Child between two angels, and a finely worked head of a man from an ancient stained glass window.

A COLLECTION OF WINE-TASTING CUPS

Somewhat startling to the visitor unacquainted with the Hospices' extensive vineyard holdings, the collection of forty silver and one wooden tastevins – wine-tasting cups – is on display in the Salle Saint-Nicolas. This is a bequest dating from 1987. While most of these items so typical of a winemaking region date from the 19th century, a dozen or so go back a further hundred years and bear the hallmarks of craftsmen from Chalon, Mâcon and Autun. The oldest of them is engraved, as custom has it, with the name of its owner: *Philippe Giboulot 1754*. The work of Gaspard Simonnot, master goldsmith in Beaune, this is a plain cup whose decorated, medallion-like thumb-rest is highly distinctive. On the 19th-century pieces we find the stamps of such other Beaune goldsmiths as Léonard Humbert and Adrien Fromageot, the latter also being the maker of a rare silver wine pipette from the same collection.

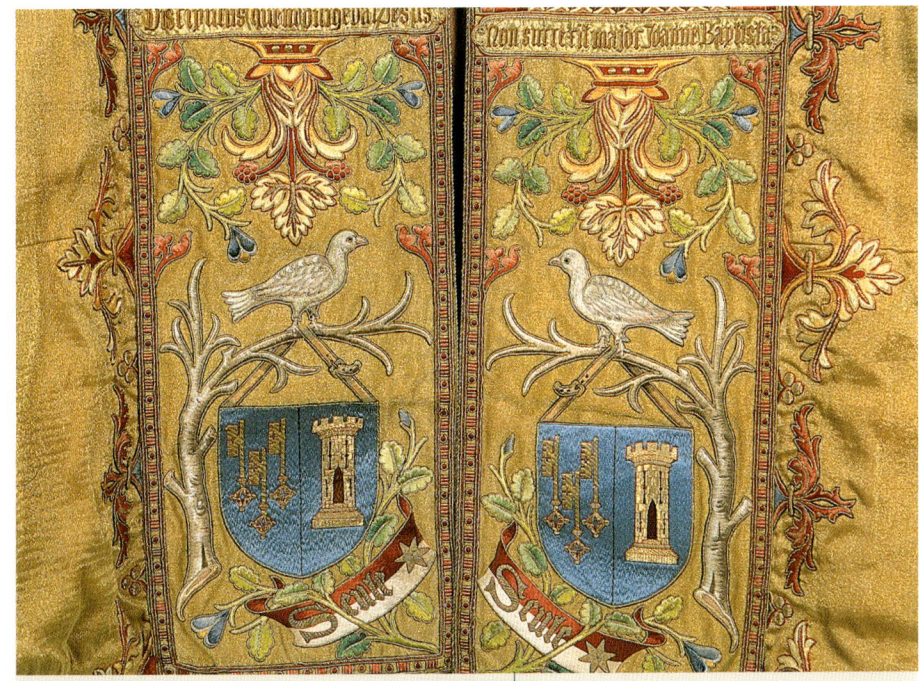

Back to the roots

The quality of the original furniture and decoration is such that ongoing restoration of the Hôtel-Dieu's buildings has led at various times to the creation of pieces directly inspired by those of the 15th century. To take an example, the three gilt oak celebrant's chairs made for the chapel in the second half of the 19th century are copies of the chair of St Peter in the *Last Judgement* polyptych. Rogier Van der Weyden's masterpiece was likewise a source of inspiration for the Dijon goldsmith Henri Dejouy, who in 1922 recreated its figures on a chalice with painted enamel embellishments.

Then there are the doves on a branch holding up a shield bearing the coat of arms of Guigone de Salins: they recur on the base of a monstrance with transparent blue enamel rays, a strikingly individual piece by Lyon goldsmith Thomas-Joseph Armand-Calliat, who worked with Viollet-le-Duc. The same motif is to be found on the embroidered orphreys of a Neo-Gothic liturgical cope.

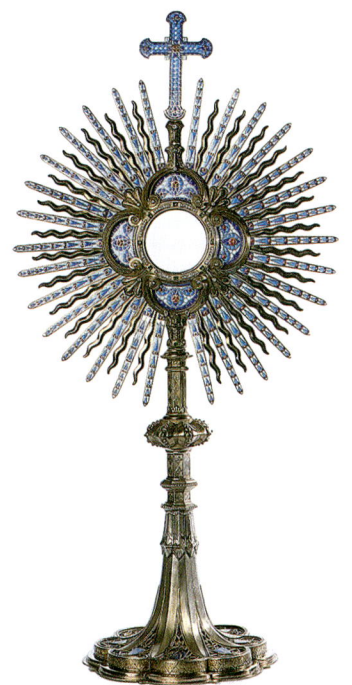

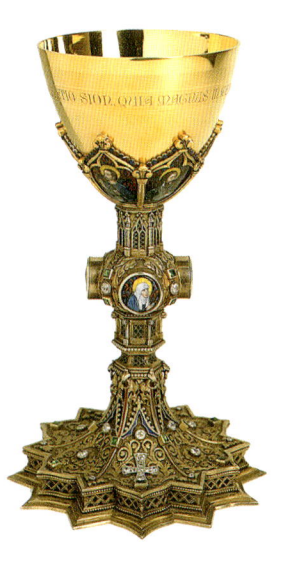

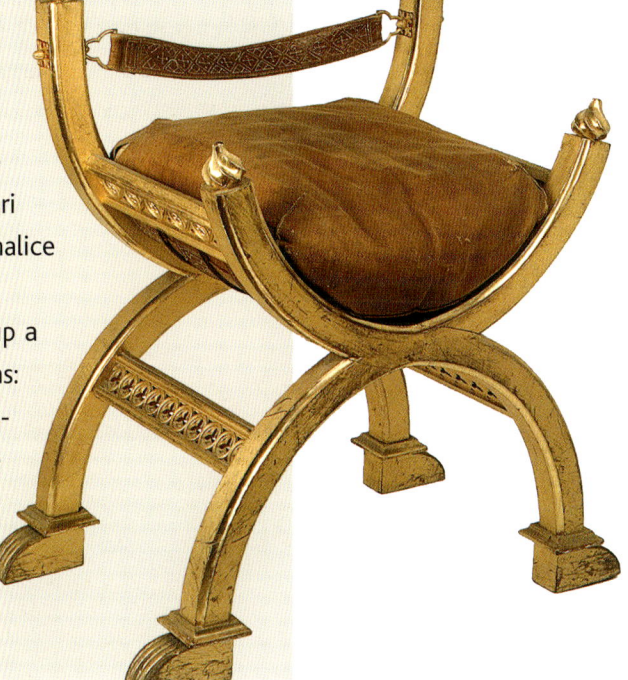

▮ Above left: Monstrance by Thomas-Joseph Armand-Calliat, second half 19th century.
Above centre: Cope (detail), second half 19th century.
Above right: Chalice by Henri Dejouy, 1922.
Lower right: Celebrant's chair, second half 19th century.

The Hospices de Beaune vineyards

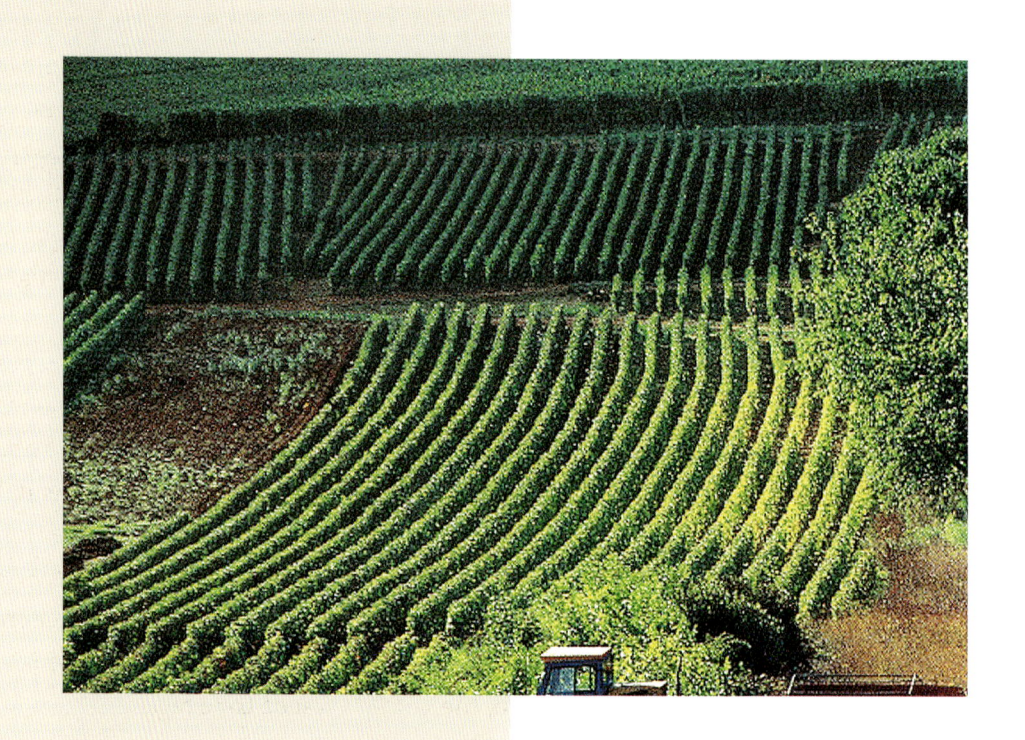

Since their establishment in 1443 the Hospices de Beaune have combined charitable works and the making of excellent wine. This is an institution that has always remained faithful to the spirit of its founder, Nicolas de Rolin, chancellor of the Duke of Burgundy: even as the Hundred Years War raged, he put his faith in future benefactors who, like himself, would show themselves generous to the very poor. This humanist philosophy has continued to flourish down the centuries, and the Hospices de Beaune have accumulated substantial assets that include their famous vineyards.

The first donation of vineyards goes back to 1457. Since then fresh legacies have gradually been added, most of them involving major vintages. Naturally enough, given the Hôtel-Dieu's location, the vineyards are mainly situated locally: at Auxey-Duresses, Beaune, Meursault, Monthelie, Pommard, Pernand-Vergelesses, Puligny-Montrachet, Savigny-lès-Beaune and Volnay. However the Hospices de Beaune also have vineyards in the Côte de Nuits, including the "grand crus" of Mazis-Chambertin and Clos de la Roche, and – since 1994 – the Mâcon area, with plots of Pouilly-Fuissé.

Totalling some 60 hectares, the vineyards are painstakingly looked after by the Hospices steward and a staff of 20 winemakers. Each winemaker is in charge of 2.5 hectares and the grapes, as elsewhere in Burgundy, are pinot noir for the red wines and chardonnay for the whites.

In the interests of impeccable quality, output is deliberately limited to 3000/3500 litres per hectare. Rigorous selection of the grapes is followed by exacting vinification ensuring that the harmony of the vintages is maintained.

The crushed red wine grapes macerate for several days in the vats while the must – a slurry of skins, juice and seeds – ferments and the tannins and colouring compounds emerge. The subsequent pressing is done pneumatically. The Hospices are no less exigent when it comes to storage. Every year the entire stock of casks is replaced with oak models from the Vosges, the forests of Tronçais and Bertranges, and the Centre-Val de Loire region.

The environment counts too, and at Beaune the natural is given priority over the chemical. The land deserves respect and a herbicide-free integrated farming approach is used.

Each of the 41 vintages represents the harmonious mix of different climates that characterises Hospices de Beaune wines. The vineyards reflect all the variety of Burgundy's best winegrowing areas and embody a tradition of meticulousness and excellence going back hundreds of years – whence the fresh spark of pleasure that comes with each tasting of these renowned *appellations*, with their generous, distinctively local characters.

The sale of Hospices de Beaune wines

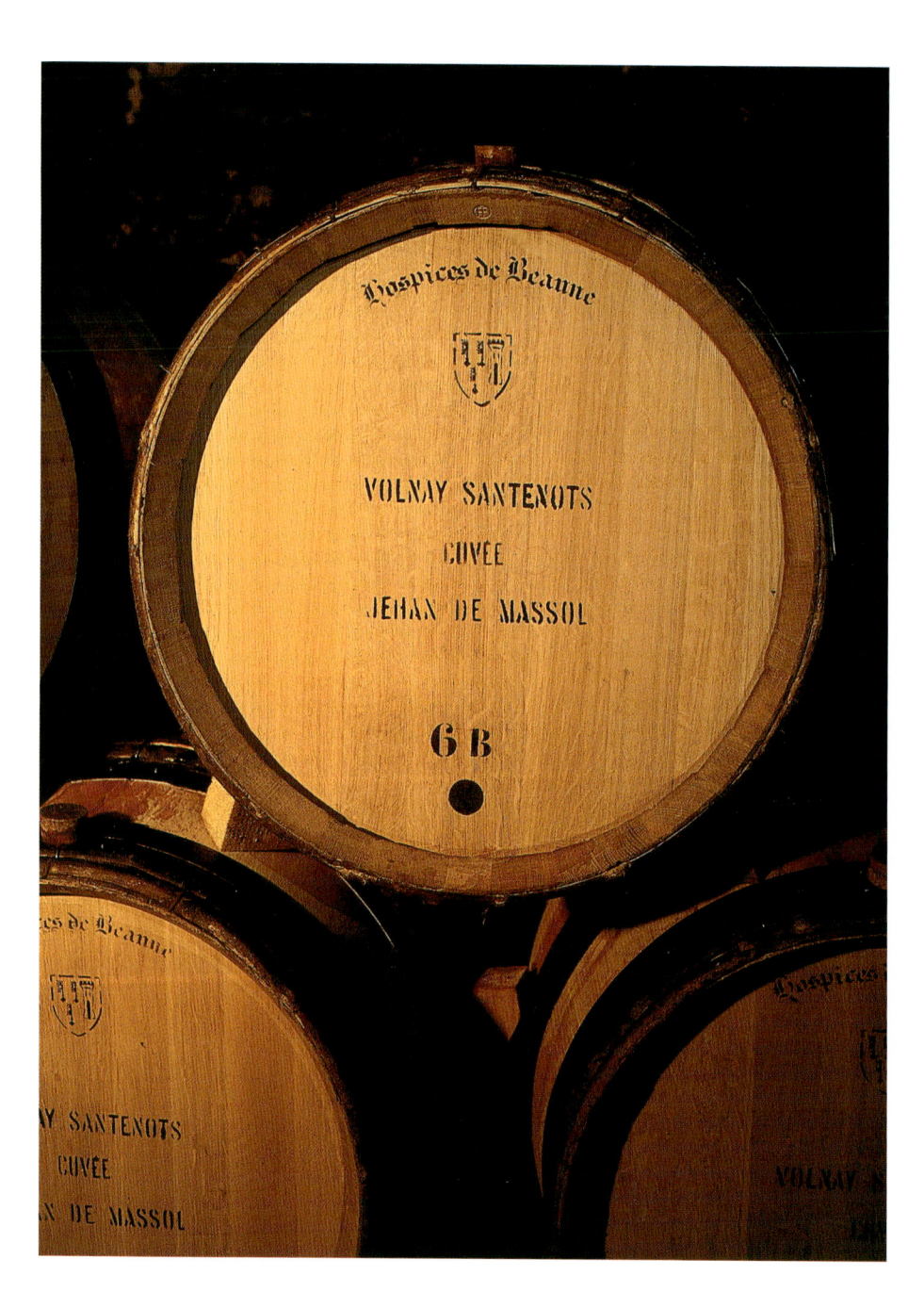

The Burgundies of Beaune were originally sold simply via advertising, but it was largely the efforts of Joseph Pétasse, winemaker, scholar and tireless ambassador for the Hospices, that brought them their reputation: he toured Europe proclaiming their virtues and quality to potential buyers, and in less than two years wine merchants had bought up the entire stock. So, free of the need to go hunting for customers, the directors held their first auction in 1859. The result: what is now the world's largest charity sale and a world-famous event eagerly awaited by wine professionals everywhere.

Until 1925 the auction was held in the main courtyard of the Hôtel-Dieu. The sale was then transferred to the fermentation cellar; and since 1959 the venue has been the covered market in Beaune;

Bidding is restricted to wine merchants from Burgundy, and private buyers can only acquire wine by using them as intermediaries. Nonetheless, the many buyers from elsewhere give the auction a truly international character.

The procedure is tried, true and unchanging. Two days before the sale come the tastings and then, on the third Sunday of November, things get under way under the eagle eye of the auctioneer. He begins with a detailed description of each lot, announces the starting price and then takes the bids as the little timing candle burns down and his assistant urges the buyers on.

As a symbol of their charitable function, each year the Hospices offer an unlisted lot. A sponsor drawn from Europe's royal families – Prince Otto of Habsburg, the Duke of Kent – or, according to a more recent custom, from the world of the arts – Barbara Hendricks, Mstistlav Rostropovich, Charlotte Rampling – is given some three hundred bottles which he or she immediately offers for sale. The proceeds are then donated to a humanitarian body of the sponsor's choice.

The prices fetched at the auctions are not an accurate reflection of current Burgundy values. On average they are two to three times higher than on the outside market: charity is the driving force of the sales and the buyers are well aware of this. Thus each participating wine merchant, like each visitor buying a ticket to watch the auction, is contributing to a worthwhile cause: the income goes towards the modernisation of medical equipment, improvements to the accommodation for the sick and aged, and the maintenance of the unique historical and cultural heritage represented by the Hôtel-Dieu.

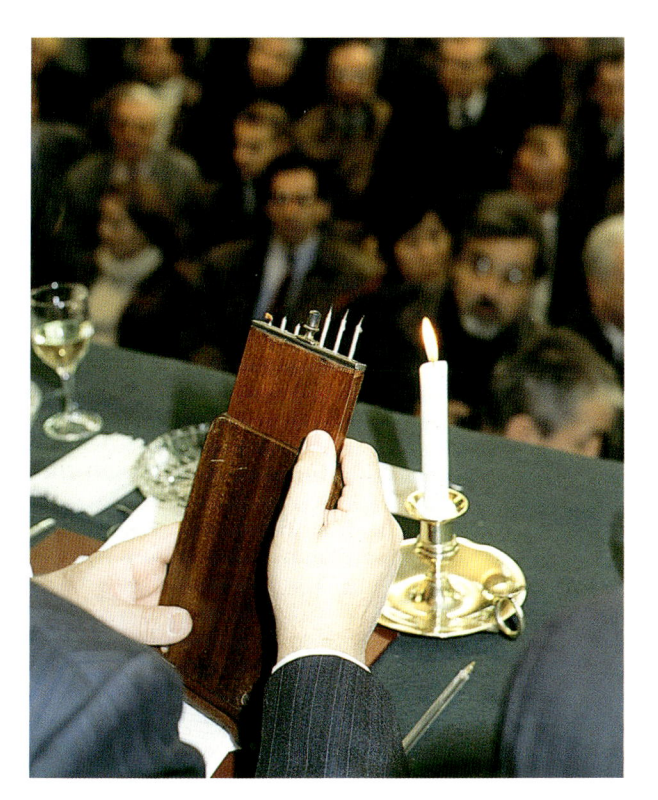

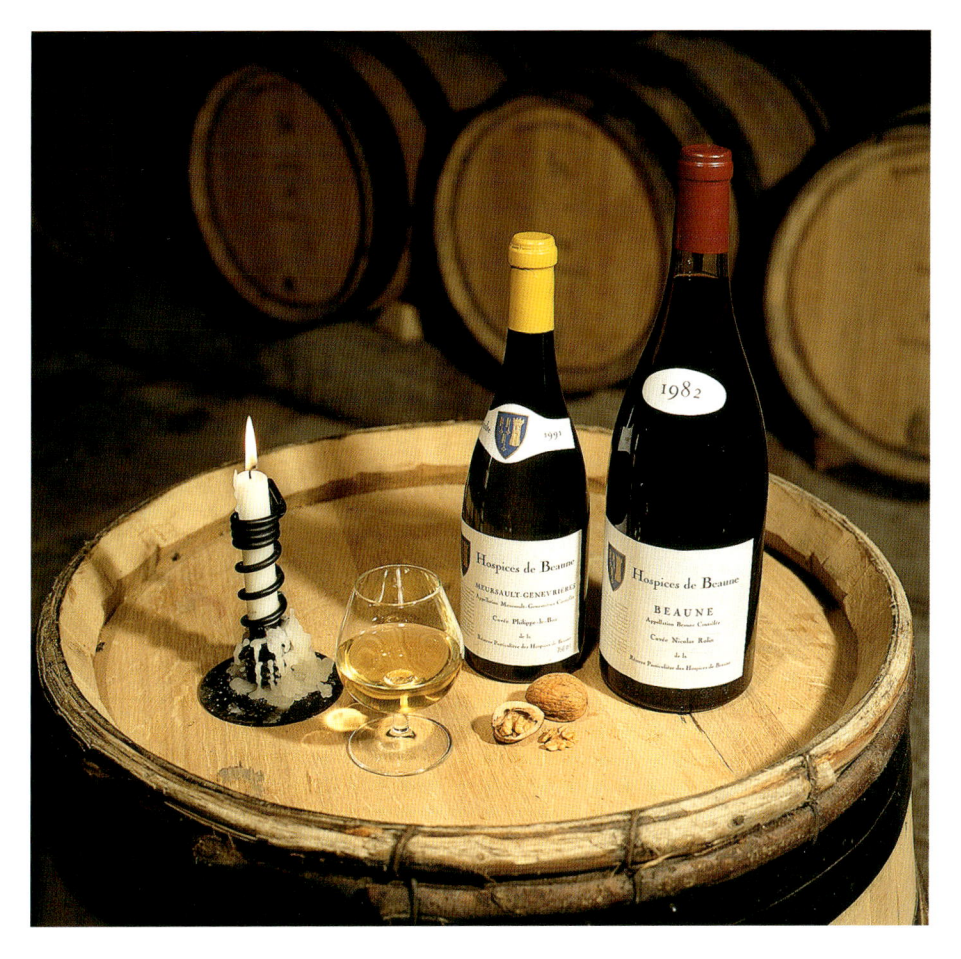

The hospital today

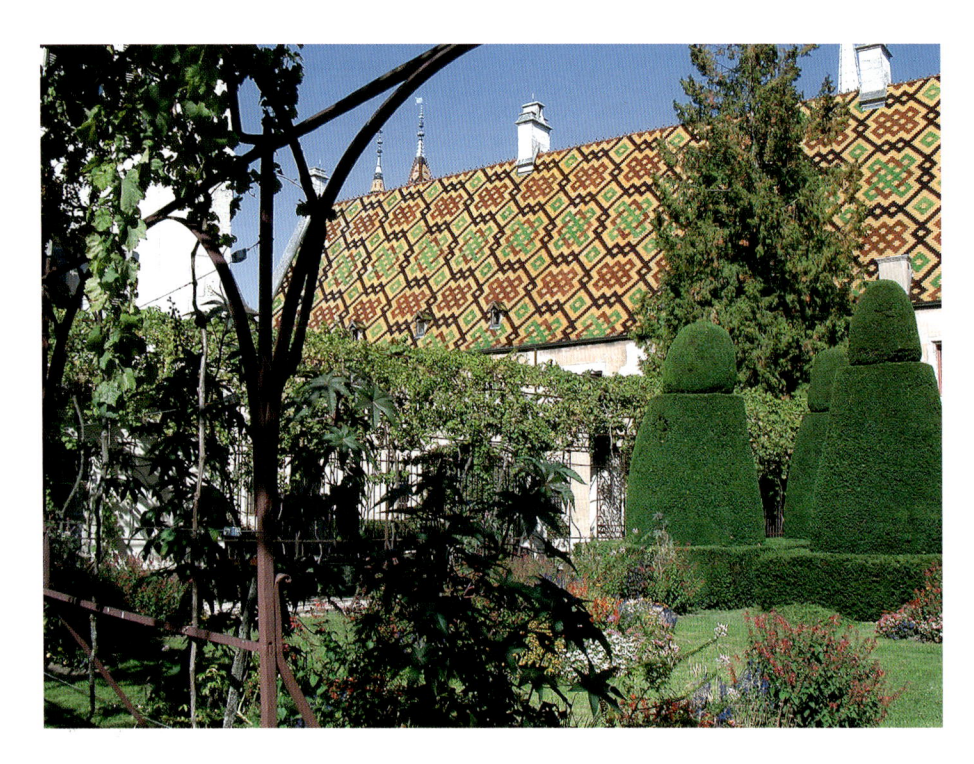

The Hospices Civils de Beaune now comprise four accommodation and treatment establishments on different sites.

The last patient to leave the Salle Saint-Hugues ward in 1983 was transferred to the Philippe-le-Bon hospital complex, the largest of these sites. Opened in 1971, it has 200 beds and ultramodern equipment, with all the departments and medicotechnical, administrative and logistic facilities needed to optimise patient care. Its emergency room is open 24 hours a day and has its own mobile intensive care unit. The complex treats some 20,000 people per year.

Established in 1984, the Nicolas Rolin Centre for the dependent aged has 90 long-stay beds and another 30 for convalescence and rehabilitation.

The Hôtel-Dieu and La Charité retirement homes offer over 170 city-centre beds in the magnificent setting of the Hôtel-Dieu itself.

In another building next to La Charité is the child guidance centre, where children in need of specialised psychological help are given ongoing individual treatment.

The Nursing Institute and the school for nursing aides offer the requisite training to those who have decided to devote themselves to the sick, in a kind of tribute to the hospitaller nuns of earlier times.

In 1993 the Hospices set up a medical care annexe for Beaune's poorest residents. Situated in the heart of the city, this facility exists to serve those unwilling to attend a hospital or see a doctor and for whom an alternative setting is required.

Today the Hôtel-Dieu is a museum whose architectural splendour, going back to the 15th century, is paralleled by the enduring yet up-to-date ethic of the hospital it gave rise to. As for all France's hospitals, running costs are covered by the Social Security system; but the extra revenue accruing from the museum and the Hospices' winemaking activity allows for added spending on the equipment, development and modernisation that ensure highly sophisticated treatment facilities.

Times change, but the tradition of help and hospitality is stronger than ever. The Hospices de Beaune remain true to the spirit of Nicolas Rolin and the mission for which they were created: to take in those in need and provide them with aid and comfort.

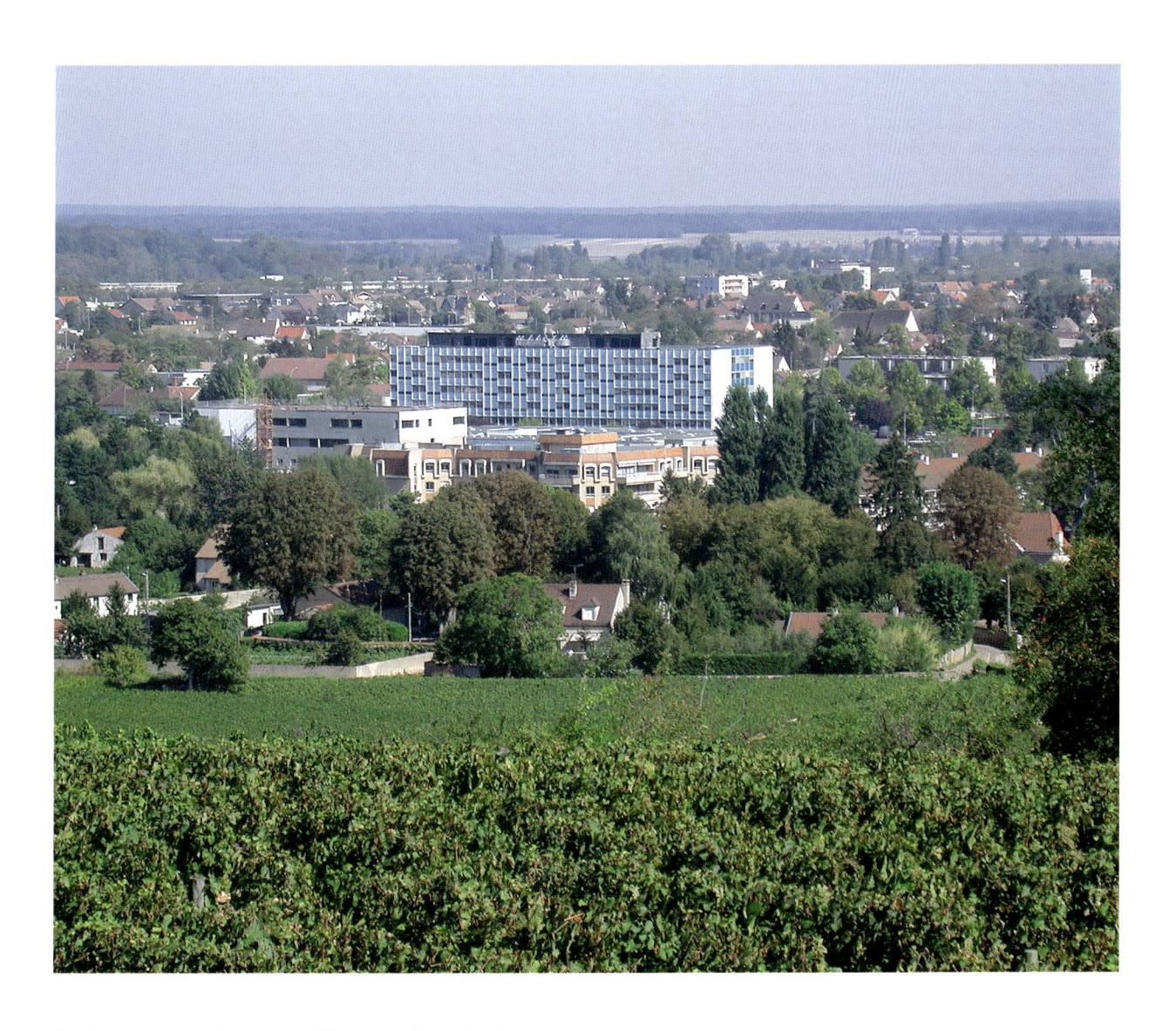

Bibliography

MANUSCRIPT SOURCES

Archives of the Department of Historical Monuments
Cartons 619-620 (1844-1987): Hôtel-Dieu. (General Inventory of the Monuments and Art Treasures of France: analytical inventory of cartons 619 and 620 from the archives of the Department of Historical Monuments, by Yves Lasfargues, 1978, typed: *City of Beaune – Charitable establishments – Hôtel-Dieu and Hospice de la Charité.*)

Archives of the Côte-d'Or département
H 1252, bundle "Beaune", file "Hôtel-Dieu", notebooks 1 and 2: building accounts of Jehannot Bar, notary and supervisor of the Hôtel-Dieu (10 June 1447-31 August 1448) [from the projected edition of Jehannot Bar's accounts, prepared by Pierre Jugie and held by the regional service of General Inventory of Burgundy].

Department of Historical Monuments, regional conservation section (current archives)
File "Beaune, Hôtel-Dieu, Restoration of the Salle Saint Nicolas", by F. Didier, 1987.

Beaune, Hôtel-Dieu archives
1. E 20-28: Register of deliberations (26 November 1631 –1er nivôse an V).
2. L 0-20: Register of deliberations (an VIII –1960).
3. E 1-3: Accounts of Jean Duban, notary and supervisor of the Hôtel-Dieu (1458-1464; 1468-1472).
4. E 2: "Memorandum of progress on new building projects begun at the Hôtel-Dieu in Beaune in 1754" (1756-1760). Unclassified archives: restoration of the Great Hall of the Poor (1845-1886); workers' records: stonecutting, masonry, roof frames, roofing, carpentry, plastering (1851-1875); plans and designs of the architect Maurice Ouradou (1872-1883).
IV O 1: works (1840-1937).
IV O 2: fermenting room (1833-1836).
IV O 23: Salle Saint-Louis and the hall of the polyptych (1972-1974).
IV O 26: modification of the Sainte-Anne pavilion, the fermenting room and the cellar (1975).

Beaune, Communal archives
H II 16: construction of the military hospital (1893-1896).

PRINTED SOURCES

Boudrot Abbé Jean-Baptiste, "Marché pour la charpente du grand corps de bâtiment sur la rue", *Mémoires de la Société d'histoire et d'archéologie de Beaune*, 1874-1875, pp. 145-150.

Boudrot Abbé Jean-Baptiste, *Petit cartulaire de l'Hostel-Dieu de Beaune. Inventaires. Bulles pontificales. Lettres patentes des ducs de Bourgogne et des rois de France*, Beaune, Batault-Morot, 1880.

SELECT BIBLIOGRAPHY

Bavard Abbé Étienne, *L'Hôtel-Dieu de Beaune (1443-1880), d'après les documents recueillis par M. l'abbé Boudrot*, Beaune, Batault-Morot, 1881.

Benoit-Cattin Renaud, "Quelques aspects de l'œuvre du peintre Isaac Moillon (1614-1673)", *In situ* (www.revue.inventaire.culture.gouv.fr), no. 2, 2000.

Cyrot Louis, "Les bâtiments du grand Hôtel-Dieu de Beaune: notice chronologique sur leur fondation et leurs accroissements d'après les archives de cet hôpital", *Mémoires de la Société d'histoire et d'archéologie de Beaune*, 1881, pp. 1-73.

FODÉRÉ Jacques, *Narration historique et topographique des Convens de l'Ordre St François, et Monastères S.-Claire, érigez en la Province anciennement appellée de Bourgongne, à présent de S.-Bonaventure,* Lyon, Pierre Rigaud, 1619.

FRANÇOIS Bruno, "Les coffres médiévaux de l'Hôtel-Dieu de Beaune: catalogue", master's thesis in medieval art and archaeology, Université de Bourgogne, U.F.R. Sciences humaines, Dijon, 1991.

FROMAGET Brigitte, REYNIÈS Nicole de, *Les Tapisseries des Hospices de Beaune,* General Inventory of the Monuments and Art Treasures of France, "Images du patrimoine" series, no. 126, Dijon, Association pour la connaissance du patrimoine de Bourgogne, 1993.

JACQUEMIN Sister, "Histoire de la règle de vie des sœurs hospitalières de Beaune", *Recueil des travaux du Centre beaunois d'études historiques,* t. 5, 1985, pp. 23-39.

JUGIE Pierre, "L'Hôtel-Dieu de Beaune", *Congrès archéologique de France, 152e session, la Côte-d'Or et la plaine de Saône, 1994,* Paris, Société française d'archéologie, 1998, pp. 203-209.

La bonne étoile des Rolin – Mécénat et efflorescence artistique dans la Bourgogne du XVe siècle, exhibition at the Musée Rolin, Beaune, Hôtel-Dieu, September-November 1994; Autun, Musée Rolin, 1994.

La Splendeur des Rolin. Un mécénat privé à la cour de Bourgogne, round table, 27-28 February 1995, Autun, Société éduenne; Paris, Picard, 1999.

Le Faste des Rolin. Au temps des ducs de Bourgogne, Dijon, Faton, "Dossiers de l'art", 49, 1998.

LOCATELLI Christine, POUSSET Didier, "Les charpentes et les lambris", dans *Vie de cour en Bourgogne à la fin du Moyen Âge*, "Histoire et archéologie" series, Saint-Cyr-sur-Loire, A. Sutton, 2002, pp. 86-98.

NAUDET abbé Henri, *La Communauté de l'Hôtel-Dieu de Beaune,* Beaune, 1934.

SÉCULA Didier, "Étude architecturale de l'Hôtel-Dieu de Beaune", postgraduate dissertation in the history of medieval art, Université de Bourgogne, Dijon, 1996. (The author's doctoral thesis was presented in 2004: "L'Hôtel-Dieu de Beaune: étude architecturale et approche iconologique d'un monument emblématique", Université de Paris IV-Sorbonne.)

SÉCULA Didier, "Le grand Hôtel-Dieu de Beaune au XVe siècle: la fondation, le personnel et les bâtiments", in *Bruges à Beaune. Marie, l'héritage de Bourgogne*, exhibition, Beaune, November 2000-February 2001; Paris, Somogy éditions d'art, Beaune, Hospices civils, 2000, pp. 141-158.

STEIN Henri, *L'Hôtel-Dieu de Beaune*, "Petites monographies des grands édifices de la France" series, Paris, 1933.

STORCK J.-Justin, *Dictionnaire pratique de menuiserie, ébénisterie, charpente*, Paris, Lardy (Seine-et-Oise), J.-J. Storck, 1899.

VERDIER Aymar, CATTOIS François, *Architecture civile et domestique au Moyen Âge et à la Renaissance*, Paris, V. Didron, 1855-1857.

VERONEE-VERHAEGHEN Nicole, " L'Hôtel-Dieu de Beaune", *Les Primitifs flamands. Corpus de la peinture des anciens Pays-Bas méridionaux au quinzième siècle*, Bruxelles, Centre national de recherches Primitifs flamands, 1973.

Photographic credits

Michel Rosso: © Inventaire général - ADAGP: pages 12, 13, 15, 16-17, 19, 20, 23, 26, 27, 29, 31, 32, 33, 35, 37, 39, 41 to 45, 49 to 51, 52 (below), 53 to 55, 58 to 61, 64, 65, 67, 69, 70-71, 73 to 77, 78-79, 81 to 85, 87, 88, 89 (right), 90, 91, 93 to 95, 96 (right), 97, 99 to 102, 105 to 117, 118 (below), 119.

Jean-Luc Duthu: © Inventaire général - ADAGP: pages 14, 24, 34, 38, 46, 48, 52 (above), 56, 57, 62, 63, 80, 89 (left), 96 (left).

Michel Thierry: © Inventaire général - ADAGP: pages 40, 66, 78 (left), 86, 103, 118 (above).

Christine Locatelli: page 25.

Hospices civils de Beaune : page 120 to 125.

Photoengraving: Quat'Coul, Toulouse.
Printed by STIGE S.P.A., April 2005.